LABTRONICS

Electronics for laboratory scientists

LABTRONICS

Electronics for laboratory scientists

L. M. Schmidt, D.A., M.T.(ASCP)

Training Development Specialist, Automatic Clinical Analysis Division,
DuPont Company, Instrument Products, Wilmington, Delaware;
Formerly Assistant Professor and Director, Medical Technology Program,
and Coordinator, Doctor of Arts in Medical Technology Program,
The Catholic University of America, Washington, D.C.; Assistant Professor
of Medical Technology, Wayne State University,
Detroit, Michigan

With **248** illustrations

The C. V. Mosby Company

ST. LOUIS · TORONTO · LONDON   1979

Cover photograph by S. A. Miller

Printed in the United States of America

The C. V. Mosby Company
11830 Westline Industrial Drive, St. Louis, Missouri 63141

Library of Congress Cataloging in Publication Data

Schmidt, L   M   1943-
   Labtronics.

   Originally presented as the author's thesis,
Catholic University of America.
   Bibliography: p.
   Includes index.
   1.   Medical laboratories—Equipment and supplies.
2. Medical electronics. 3. Medical technologists.
I. Title. [DNLM: 1. Electronics, Medical. QT34.3
S353L5]
RB110.2.S3   1979   621.381   78-31415
ISBN 0-8016-4342-2

C/M/M 9 8 7 6 5 4 3 2 1   03/0/301

To the memory of
Emil Schmidt

PREFACE

Instruments used in clinical laboratories are increasing in number, variety, and sophistication. In the performance of analytical procedures, electronic circuits have replaced the manual manipulations of yesteryear. Therefore, to keep pace, laboratory scientists must learn the language and the fundamental principles of this new generation of laboratory equipment.

Laboratory scientists are required to calibrate, operate, maintain, and trouble-shoot analytical instruments used in clinical laboratories. Limited knowledge of basic electronics seriously handicaps scientists in the effective performance of these functions. Therefore, the intent of this book is to provide laboratory science students with an understanding of the major concepts of electronics, the function of electronic components in various circuit configurations, and the applicability of these concepts and components to the operational principles of analytical instruments. Students should develop a keen awareness of requisite automatic and adjustable electronic responses of properly functioning instruments. Only after students are able to predict and recognize normal functions of a circuit or an instrument can they identify and evaluate malfunctions. This book will not train students to be expert troubleshooters of circuits or instruments, but it will provide the first step in establishing an appreciation of the interrelatedness of electrical concepts, electronic components, and operational theories of analytical instruments.

This book presents overall concepts and principles of electronics through simplified explanations and figures rather than mathematical proofs. A year of college general physics more than adequately provides the prerequisite knowledge for using this book.

The book is divided into five sections. Section One includes a discussion of the six basic functional units of analytical instruments. This section provides a point of reference for establishing a relationship between electronics and instruments. This link between instrumentation and electronics is reinforced throughout the text in two ways. First, clinical laboratory instruments are used as examples for illustrating or clarifying applications of electronic principles. Second, Section Four discusses functional units of analytical instruments, applying facts, concepts, and principles presented in Sections Two and Three. Section Two, Fundamentals of Electronics, presents the concept of electricity and the parameters associated with it, such as voltage, current, resistance, and power. Direct current, alternating current, and circuit configurations are also discussed. Section Three includes relatively detailed discussions of electronic components: resistors, capacitors, inductors, transformers, and diodes. The detail of this section is justified by the fact that electronic components are the building blocks of circuits, simple or complex. Section Five deals with electrical safety and offers a stepwise approach to troubleshooting.

The book is organized to provide, when applicable, learning experiences and exercises at the ends of chapters. The instructional activities can be used by the instructor as demonstrations or laboratory projects. The practice problems and study questions should be completed by students using the text. An increased understanding of principles and a capacity for self-evaluation of comprehension of a chapter's material are benefits derived from effort applied to problem solving. Self-evaluation is made possible because students are provided with problem solutions and their derivations.

This book began to develop as lecture notes for a basic electronics course in the Medical Technology Department at Wayne State University and ended as an instructional unit accepted as a dissertation for the Doctor of Arts degree at The Catholic University of America. Invaluable contributions toward the development of this book were the administrative support provided by Dorothy M. Skinner, the unlimited access to the technical expertise and the electronics laboratory of Dr. Yeong W. Kim, and the critical evaluations of each of four manuscript revisions and the continued encouragement of Dr. Isobel Rutherford. Suggestions and comments offered by Dr. John B. Hunt, Dr. Eugene R. Kennedy, Dr. Jerry H. Roberts, and Dr. Francis X. Powell were valuable in the final manuscript revision. The generosity with which these professionals gave their time, effort, and expertise to assist in the development of this text is commendable, and I gratefully acknowledge their contributions.

L. M. Schmidt

CONTENTS

Introduction

During the performance of qualitative and/or quantitative automated procedures, an instrument operator can be a slave or a master. To be a slave is the easier and perhaps the more popular of the two choices. Samples are placed in the well labeled "sample well." A glowing "start" button is pushed. The "read" switch is thrown. A sounding alarm indicates malfunction, and illuminated immediately is the telephone number of the nearest service representative. Thus the flashing lights, buzzing alarms, numbered buttons, and driving gears lead, direct, and essentially command the ordered manipulations to be performed on the instrument by its assigned servant. Unhappiness does not necessarily plague this instrument operator who, in the bliss for which ignorance has been credited, believes himself or herself to be in control.

To be master over the instrument is a position not to be bought, scheduled, bestowed, or pretended but rather to be earned through study and application. Study and comprehension of operational principles of instrumentation provide the knowledge required for making judgments. Many decisions must be made in establishing a preventive maintenance schedule and a parts supply, in recognizing and repairing instrument malfunctions, and in selecting, designing, and executing an effective mode of instruction for instrument operators.

During the operation of a properly functioning instrument, there is no apparent difference between the slave and the master. However, this appearance is the end of the similarity. The master *is* in control. Pushing a button or throwing a switch is accompanied by the ability to intelligently interpret the effect each such manipulation has on instrument functions. As a result, less than optimal instrument performance may be accepted obliviously by the slave but will be perceived keenly by the master.

It is naive to think that knowledge of instrumental principles will transform a laboratory analyst into a troubleshooting wizard capable of pinpointing and repairing all instrumental deficiencies. This is certainly not the case. The operator of analytical instruments should be able to recognize when an instrument is not functioning properly, identify the problem, and evaluate the availability of resources required for repair. If parts are at hand for a minor repair, an individual capable of performing this repair could do so. Immediate repair could avoid expenditure of the time, the money, and the effort needed to implement a back-up method. However, if instrument malfunction diagnosis or repair is problematic, expert assistance should be requested. Of utmost importance is the ability to evaluate both the extent of an instrumental problem and the extent of one's own capabilities to rectify the problem. It is better to keep hands off than to approach a malfunctioning instrument with irresponsible overconfidence.

Confidence derived from knowledge of instrumental principles is required for the analyst to control and operate analytical instruments. These instruments are made up of functional units, the majority of which are electronic. Electronic units are composed of an assortment of electronic devices, such as resistors, capacitors, diodes, transistors, operational amplifiers, transformers, choppers, inductors, switches, and potentiometers. It is, therefore, difficult to comprehend principles of analytical instruments without first having a basic vocabulary and a fundamental understanding of electronic devices and their functional principles.

The purpose of this text is to provide a foundation of knowledge in basic electronics relevant to the functional principles of analytical instruments. To link the abstract to the concrete, this book will apply the theoretical principles of electronics to the functional units of instruments. Six basic functional units of analytical instruments can serve as a tangible framework to which electronic principles can be related. These six functional units, as shown in Fig. 1-1, are the power source, the excitation or signal source, the sample compartment, the detector, the signal processing unit, and the readout device. Each of these units will be described briefly in this introductory section.

CHAPTER 1

BASIC FUNCTIONAL UNITS
OF ANALYTICAL INSTRUMENTS

The basic functional units of analytical instruments, as shown in Fig. 1-1, are the power source, the excitation or signal source, the sample compartment, the detector, the signal processing unit, and the readout device.

SAMPLE COMPARTMENT

The sample compartment is described first because it is the functional unit with which laboratory scientists are most familiar. The sample compartment holds the sample to be analyzed. Delivery of the sample into the sample compartment occurs after the sample has been prepared according to instrument and methodology requirements. The sample form required for analysis may be gaseous, liquid, or solid. Gas chromatographs and mass spectrophotometers, for example, quantitatively analyze gaseous samples. Spectrophotometers, emission flame photometers, atomic absorption spectrophotometers, osmometers, pH meters, titrators, and automatic cell counters analyze liquid samples. Solid samples can be analyzed with electron microscopes and x-ray spectrometers.

POWER SOURCE

The power source supplies power to all electrical units of the instrument. Batteries and commercially generated power supplies are two sources of power.

Batteries generate direct current as a product of electrochemical reactions. They are not generally used as the sole source of power in analytical instruments

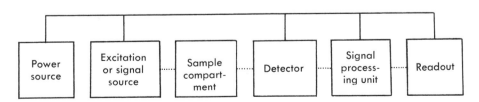

Fig. 1-1. Basic functional units of analytical instruments. Electrical connections from the power source are indicated by solid lines. Physical and/or electrical interconnections between units are designated by dotted lines.

but occasionally are used within a particular circuit of an instrument to perform a specific function. Use of batteries as a power source is limited because they are heavy, may be destructive if caustic agents leak into an instrument, and may be expensive and troublesome since replacements are required. However, they do provide the advantage of portability. If instrumental analyses are needed in locations not accessible to electrical generators, battery operated instruments can be used.

The diversified power requirements of instrument circuits are in most cases fulfilled by a power supply. Commercially generated alternating current is fed from a wall power outlet through a power cord into an instrument's power supply. The electrical needs of each component within an instrument are not necessarily the same. One component may require alternating current (ac), while another may require direct current (dc). Requirements for regulation of voltage, current, and stability also may differ from one component to another. The power supply must fulfil the specific electrical requirement of each electronic unit. Therefore, the power supply must:

1. *Transform* ac voltage to higher and/or lower voltages than the 115 volts ac (Vac) input voltage
2. *Rectify* alternating current to direct current
3. *Regulate* the stability of direct current to meet the specified requirements of dc-operated components (Electronic drift within an instrument's circuit could result in erroneous readout signals and incorrect test results.)

EXCITATION OR SIGNAL SOURCE

Sample analyses are performed by instruments that expose the sample to some type of energy. Quantification of a constituent within a sample can be accomplished by measuring the effect the sample constituent has on a preset energy signal or the effect certain energy has on the physical and/or chemical properties of the sample constituent.

The sample may cause a measurable change in an energy signal. In spectrophotometry, a light signal is detected and measured. A sample is then placed between the light source and the detector, causing the amount of light hitting the detector to be diminished. The change in the amount of light reaching the detector before and after sample introduction is related to the concentration of a radiant-energy–absorbing constituent in the sample.

An electrical potential may be used as a signal source as in the coulometric titration of chloride. A steady current is applied between two silver generator electrodes immersed in a sample containing chloride. The current causes constant generation of silver ions into the sample solution. Silver ions combine with chloride ions until all the chloride has precipitated as silver chloride and an excess of silver ion is generated. This excess of silver ions increases the conductivity of the solution. With increased conductivity, the current between the two indicator electrodes increases to a preset level that turns off a timer. The time required for excess silver ions to be detected as an increase in conductivity is related to chloride concentration.

An excitation source may change a property of the sample. This change may be physically or electronically measured and related to the concentration of a sample constituent. An example of an excitation source is the flame in an emission flame photometer. Heat from the flame excites atoms from their unexcited ground state to a higher energy level. As the atoms return to their original ground state, light is emitted. The emitted light can be used to identify and quantitate elements in a sample. Excitation of a sample can be caused by various forms of energy, including heat and light (for example, in fluorometry).

DETECTOR

The function of the detector is to generate an analog signal (electrical signal) from energy derived from the signal source or from an excited, electrochemically active sample.

A transducer is a detector that changes one form of energy into another form. Generally the detectors in analytical instruments convert chemical or physical energy (for example, pressure, temperature, and light) into an electrical signal. Chemical properties of a blood sample are detected for blood gas and blood pH determinations. The pH is determined by an electrode that converts hydrogen ion activity into an electrical signal. Two examples of physical signals used in analytical instruments and their transducers are:

1. Light (spectrophotometer, emission flame photometer, atomic absorption spectrophotometer, and flurometer): Transducers used for converting light to an electrical signal include barrier-layer cells, phototubes, and photomultiplier tubes.
2. Temperature (freezing point depression osmometer): A thermistor reflects a change of temperature as a change in an electrical signal.

SIGNAL PROCESSING UNIT

The detector generates an electrical signal that must be converted into understandable data related to concentration of a sample constituent for display on the readout device. This conversion is executed by the signal processing unit. This signal processing unit may be simple or complex, depending upon the sophistication of the instrument. In most cases, the signal from the detector is amplified before being fed into the readout device. Several functions performed by signal processing electronics are:

1. Signal amplification
2. Conversion of current to voltage
3. Comparison of signal to reference signal
4. Division of one signal by another
5. Addition or subtraction of two signals
6. Logarithmic conversion of signal
7. Zero adjustment
8. Calibration
9. Conversion of analog to digital signal
10. Integration and/or differentiation of signal

READOUT DEVICE

The readout device presents in visible form data obtained from sample analyses. These data should be easily read and understood. In most analytical instruments, the output data represent concentrations of specific sample constituents. The readout device in a sense translates the electrical signals from the detector and the signal processing electronics into physical or concentration values. The most frequently seen readout devices on clinical analytical instruments include:

1. Meter
2. Digital display
3. Recorder
4. Print-out
5. Cathode ray tube

FROM THE GENERAL TO THE SPECIFIC

The general view of instruments' functional units can be applied to specific instruments to allow for quick, logical modular disassembly into comprehensible working units. The student of instrumentation should practice identifying the six basic functional units of instruments. At the end of this chapter is a section of instructional activities to which the student should refer for additional learning experiences.

This brief overview of the building blocks of instruments will now serve as the portal through which the material in the following chapters will be viewed. Knowledge of electronic concepts, components, modules, and rules of safety will strengthen theoretical and practical proficiency in instrumentation.

INSTRUCTIONAL ACTIVITIES

1. Students are instructed in the operational procedures and theories of specific instruments. Instruction may be given in a variety of forms, for example, demonstrations, lectures, or reading assignments. Students are then asked to identify the basic functional units of each instrument studied. Each functional unit's specific roles within a specified instrument should also be discussed by the student.
   Examples: a. Spectrophotometer (with 700 nm to 400 nm wavelength range)
             b. Emission flame photometer

   a. Basic functional units of a spectrophotometer

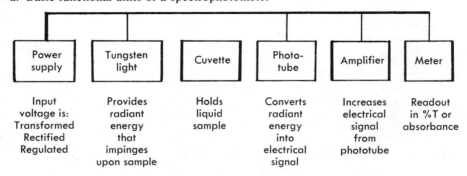

b. Basic functional units of an emission flame photometer

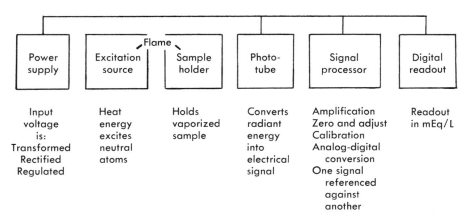

2. Students are asked to name and list specific functions performed by the basic functional units of two instruments with which they are familiar.

Fundamentals of electronics

Fundamental to knowledge of electronics is an understanding of terms. The establishment of a basic electronics vocabulary is essential for an appreciation of electronic concepts and principles. In this section, electricity is defined in terms of the interrelated parameters of current, voltage, resistance, and power. Conductors and insulators are described in terms of the atomic structures of materials. Sources and characteristics of direct and alternating current are briefly discussed.

CHAPTER 2

BASIC CONCEPTS OF ELECTRICITY

Comprehension of electrical principles begins with an understanding of the structure of the atom, which determines the availability of moveable charges. Atoms of insulators restrict movement of electrical charges, while those of conductors allow easy passage when electromotive force is applied to a closed circuit. Current, voltage, and resistance are interdependent electrical parameters, their interrelatedness being expressed in Ohm's law. Voltage drop, voltage division, power, and electrical grounding are important fundamental electronic concepts. The definitions and principles presented in this chapter are prerequisite to developing a basic understanding of what is happening in electric circuits.

THE ATOM

A discussion of electricity must begin somewhere, and the most logical starting point is the atom. The atom is the basic building block of all matter, including the matter of understanding electricity. Details of atomic structure have been studied in prerequisite chemistry and physics courses. Therefore, atomic structure will be mentioned only briefly and from the point of view applicable to electricity.

Described simply, the atom includes: (1) a *nucleus* made up of positively charged *protons* and uncharged *neutrons* and (2) negatively charged *electrons* that revolve in fixed orbits around the nucleus. The negative charge of an electron is exactly equal to the positive charge of a proton. An atom with an equal number of protons and electrons is electrically neutral. If an atom loses an electron, a proton excess—or more accurately, an electron deficiency—results. This atom carries a positive charge and is called a positive *ion*. If the atom gains an electron, the atom carries a negative charge and is called a negative ion.

Electrons in the outermost shell of the atom have a weaker attraction to the nucleus than electrons in any of the closer shells. It is these outer-shell electrons that can be freed most easily from the atom. Thermal, radiant, physical, or chemical energy applied to the atom may act as the force required to liberate one or more electrons from the outer shell. Free charges moving about suggests electricity—that is, the capacity for electron flow. Thus the outermost shell of the atom is recognized as the orbit most important in electronics.

Most metals are made up of atoms with loosely bound electrons in the outer shells. These electrons may be so loosely bound that they are constantly moving randomly from one atom to another. Picture a metal wire in which many electrons are moving about aimlessly. These electrons can be made to move in one direction by placing an excess of electrons (negative charge) at one end of the wire and a deficiency of electrons (positive charge) at the other end. The loose electrons in the wire will be repelled by the extra electrons entering the wire at the negative end and attracted to the positive charge at the other end. This electron flow is diagramed in Fig. 2-1. A stepwise description of what is happening in the wire follows:

1. An electron is introduced at the negative end of the wire.
2. This electron replaces a loose electron in an atom.
3. The now free electron is repelled by the newly introduced electron and moves to another atom.
4. Here it replaces another loose electron, repels this replaced electron, and moves on.
5. This chain reaction continues until the extra electron reaches the other end of the wire, where it is accepted by a positively charged atom.

The process as described above may sound slow, but it occurs at the speed of light (approximately 186,000 miles per second).

CONDUCTORS AND INSULATORS

Materials composed of atoms with weakly bound electrons in the outer orbits make good pathways for electron flow. Such materials are called *conductors*. The more loosely bound the outer electrons of the atoms of a material, the better the material is as a conductor (for example, silver is the best conductor, followed by copper and gold).

A nonconductor, or *insulator*, is a material in which the electrons in the outer shells of the atoms are held very tightly in their orbits. These electrons are not free to move; therefore, an electric current is unable to pass through this material. Examples of insulators include glass, plastic, and rubber.

Solids are conductors or insulators in varying degrees. What about solutions? Pure water is a relatively poor conductor but nevertheless does conduct electricity. If sodium chloride is added to pure water, the solution becomes a better conductor. When the salt is dissolved, the sodium becomes a positively charged ion (Na^+) and the chloride becomes a negatively charged ion (Cl^-). These charges will conduct electricity through the solution. The numbers and types of ions present in solution determine the conducting capacity, or conductivity, of that solution.

ELECTROMOTIVE FORCE

In order for electron flow to occur, a good conducting material must serve as an unbroken pathway for electrons, and an electron excess and an electron deficit must be applied at opposite ends of the conducting pathway.

The conducting material has already been discussed. Unresolved is the source of the electron excess and the electron deficit that are applied to opposite ends

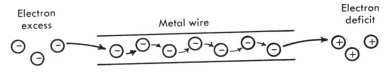

Fig. 2-1. Electron flow through a metal wire.

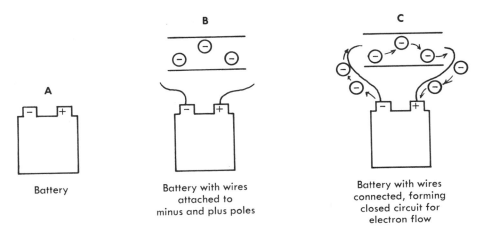

Fig. 2-2. Battery providing electromotive force for electron flow.

of a conducting wire to initiate and maintain the flow of electrons. As shown in Fig. 2-1, it appears as though the excess electrons are pushing or forcing the free or loose electrons through the wire. In fact, this process *is* regarded as a *force*. The force exerted by the excess electrons upon the loose electrons in the conductor is quite appropriately called *electromotive force* (EMF). The electromotive force is the *force* that causes *electrons* to *move* through a conductor from a negatively to a positively charged point. The unit of measure of electromotive force is the *volt*. (The definition of the volt will be presented later in this chapter.)

What supplies this electromotive force? Some type of battery or generator may be the source of the required EMF. A *battery* is a direct current voltage source consisting of cells that convert one form of energy (chemical, thermal, nuclear, or solar) to electrical energy. An ac *generator* is an alternating current voltage source consisting of a rotating mechanism that converts mechanical energy into electrical energy.

The batteries with which we are most familiar convert chemical energy to electrical energy. Different types of batteries will be discussed in Chapter 3. Through a chemical reaction, an electron excess is formed at one pole (negative pole) and an electron deficit at the other pole (positive pole). Refer to Fig. 2-2. As shown in this figure, if the positive and negative poles of a battery are connected with a conducting material, electrons will flow from the negative pole to the positive pole. The battery therefore provides the force (EMF) required to move the electrons through the conductor. Fig. 2-3 is the same as Fig. 2-2, but the conventional schematic symbols are used.

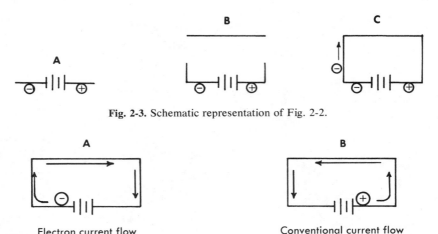

Fig. 2-3. Schematic representation of Fig. 2-2.

Electron current flow   Conventional current flow

Fig. 2-4. Electrical current flow.

CURRENT

It has been established that electrons can be forced to flow through a conductor. Now relate this electron flow to electrical current. Refer to Fig. 2-4. The circuit in *A* represents electron flow from negative to positive. Traditionally, however, current has been thought to flow from positive to negative, as represented in Fig. 2-4, *B*. This concept is considered the conventional way of perceiving current flow. In the literature both concepts of current flow may be found. Throughout this text the conventional current flow, positive to negative, will be used.

Current (designated I) is the rate at which a *charge* moves through a conductor. What is a charge? Each electron possesses energy called a charge (designated Q). The unit for measuring this charge is the *coulomb* (abbreviated C). Each electron carries an approximate charge of 1.6×10^{-19} C. How many electrons would it take to accumulate a charge of 1 C? The charges of 6,240,000,000,000,000,000 electrons added together would give a charge of 1 C. Therefore, 1 C equals 6.24×10^{18} electrons.

The unit of measure of current is the *ampere* (abbreviated A). When 6.24×10^{18} electrons (one coulomb) pass a point in the circuit every second, the circuit is said to be carrying a current of one ampere. For example, if the rate of flow of the electrons is 3.12×10^{18} electrons (0.5 C) per second, the current is 0.5 A. The ampere is a rather large unit. In most cases the current in circuits is in the milliampere (mA) or the microampere (μA) range. A milliampere equals one thousandth or 0.001 of an ampere, and a microampere equals one millionth or 0.000001 of an ampere.

Current is the rate of electron flow in a circuit. Two factors that affect this rate of flow are: (1) the force, or *voltage,* that moves the electrons through the circuit and (2) the ease with which the material in the circuit allows the electrons to pass, or in other words, the *resistance* of the circuit to current flow. Current and the two factors affecting it are interdependent phenomena. In the following discussion of the two factors, keep in mind that one cannot be defined without consideration of the other. These factors will now be considered separately.

VOLTAGE

The force that moves electrons through a conductor is the electromotive force. The unit of measure of EMF is the volt (V). A force of one volt is required to move one coulomb per second (one ampere) through a resistance (R) of one ohm (indicated with the Greek letter omega: Ω). Commonly used units of voltage include the kilovolt (kV), which equals 1000 volts; the megavolt (MV), 1,000,000 volts; the millivolt (mV), 0.001 volt; and the microvolt (μV), 0.000001 volt.

Electromotive force, voltage, and potential or potential difference are terms frequently used interchangeably. There are, however, subtle differences that should be noted. In the case shown in Fig. 2-2, *B,* the circuit is not closed; therefore, no electrons are moving in the conductor. No voltage is developed. However, a *potential* for current flow does exist because there are two poles of different charges, or it may be said that between the two poles there exists a *potential difference.* In Fig. 2-2, *C* the circuit is closed, and there is a voltage or EMF forcing a current to flow.

RESISTANCE

If a material is a poor conductor of electricity, it will offer resistance to current flow in a circuit. Resistance (R) to current is measured in *ohms* (Ω). The kilohm (kΩ) is one thousand ohms. The megohm (MΩ) is one million ohms. One ohm is the value of resistance through which one volt maintains a current of one ampere. The schematic symbol for resistance in a circuit is ——/\/\/\/\——. The types and construction of resistors will be presented later during the discussion of electronic components.

What is meant by "drawing current"? If a fixed potential exists, such as in a battery, the amount of current that will flow in a closed circuit of conducting material depends upon the ease with which electrons are allowed to move through the circuit. That is, if the excess electrons provided by the battery have difficulty in getting through the circuit, very few will be persistent enough to make the trip from one pole to the other. This is the case when the circuit contains high resistance. Electron flow will be very small. On the other hand, when the road is easy, many electrons will take to travel. With decreased or small resistance, there is a large current. Therefore, a circuit with little resistance draws a larger current than a circuit with large resistance.

OHM'S LAW

The relationship of voltage, current, and resistance is expressed in Ohm's law:

Voltage = current × resistance

or:

Volts = amperes × ohms

or:

$$E = I \times R$$

Solving for I:

$$I = E/R$$

Solving for R:

$$R = E/I$$

Voltage, current, and resistance and their interrelationships can be further explained or clarified by using an analogy to which all automobile operators will be able to relate—traffic. Think of each car as a bundle of 6.24×10^{18} electrons or as a charge of 1 C. The roads are conductors. Any degree of road blockage is a resistor. The more cars waiting to enter a roadway, the higher the potential for traffic flow (current) on that roadway.

Suppose a traffic light regulates traffic so well that there are always 10 cars waiting on the entrance ramp at the beginning of a two-lane roadway. When there is no work being done on the road, traffic flows over a counting device at 10 cars per second. Arbitrarily call the normal resistance to traffic flow 1. Now suppose that one of the two lanes is closed. Resistance to traffic flow therefore is doubled to 2.

Traffic flow before road work:

$$I = \text{Potential/resistance}$$
$$\text{Traffic flow} = 10 \text{ cars}/1 = 10 \text{ cars/second}$$

Traffic flow after road block:

$$\text{Traffic flow} = 10 \text{ cars}/2 = 5 \text{ cars/second}$$

This demonstrates that, with a constant potential for traffic flow, a change in resistance will affect that flow. The same is true of current flow in an electrical circuit.

VOLTAGE DROP AND VOLTAGE DIVISION

Voltage has been defined as the force required to push a current through a resistance. When the current goes through this resistance, energy is given off in the form of heat. This loss of energy can be regarded as a loss of voltage or as a *voltage drop*. Frequently voltage drop is referred to as IR drop. There is no difference in these terms, since voltage = $I \times R$. Refer to Fig. 2-5. The voltage at point *a* is 3 V, which is supplied by a 3 V battery. The voltage at point *b* is 0 V, since 3 V were dropped or lost in going through the resistor.

The concept of voltage drop may be, and frequently is, used to obtain different voltages from one voltage source. In other words, it is possible to divide a voltage source into smaller voltage sources. This is called *voltage division*. How is this done? Refer to Fig. 2-6, *A*. The circuit shown has a 3 V battery and three 1 kΩ resistors. Three volts is dropped across three resistors of equal value. The voltage at point *a* is 3 V, and the voltage at point *d* is 0 V. Since each of the three

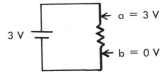

Fig. 2-5. Voltage drop.

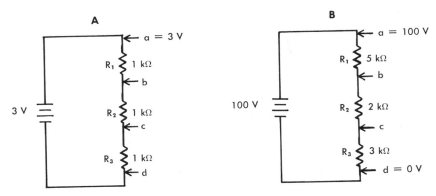

Fig. 2-6. Voltage division.

resistors will exert the same resistance to current flow, the voltage lost in each resistor will be the same. Thus 1 V is lost across each resistor. With reference to the negative side of the battery, determine the voltage readings at points *b* and *c*.

Point $b = 2$ V and point $c = 1$ V.

Voltage division is not always done by using resistors of equal value. A voltage may be dropped across any number of different resistances. The amount of voltage lost across a given resistor can be calculated in two ways:

1. Multiply the total voltage by the fraction that the given resistor is of the total resistance. For example, referring to Fig. 2-6, *B*, calculate the voltage lost across each resistor:

Total resistance $(R_t) = R_1 + R_2 + R_3$
$$R_t = 5 \text{ k}\Omega + 2 \text{ k}\Omega + 3 \text{ k}\Omega = 10 \text{ k}\Omega$$
Voltage drop in R_1: IR drop $= 100 \text{ V} \times R_1/R_t = 100 \text{ V} \times 5 \text{ k}\Omega/100 \text{ k}\Omega = 50$ V
Voltage drop in R_2: IR drop $= 100 \text{ V} \times R_2/R_t = 100 \text{ V} \times 2 \text{ k}\Omega/10 \text{ k}\Omega = 20$ V
Voltage drop in R_3: IR drop $= 100 \text{ V} \times R_3/R_t = 100 \text{ V} \times 3 \text{ k}\Omega/10 \text{ k}\Omega = 30$ V

2. Multiply total current (in amperes) passing through the resistor by the value of the resistor (in ohms). For example, referring to Fig. 2-6, *B*, calculate the voltage lost across each resistor:

Total current $(I_t) = V/R_t = 100 \text{ V}/10 \text{ k}\Omega = 10$ mA or 0.01 A
Voltage drop in R_1: IR drop $= I \times R = (0.01 \text{ A}) (5,000 \text{ }\Omega) = 50$ V
Voltage drop in R_2: IR drop $= I \times R = (0.01 \text{ A}) (2,000 \text{ }\Omega) = 20$ V
Voltage drop in R_3: IR drop $= I \times R = (0.01 \text{ A}) (3,000 \text{ }\Omega) = 30$ V

The application of voltage division will be seen frequently throughout the remainder of this text. It is very important that this basic concept be understood at this time.

POWER

Another term to be considered is power. When electrons are pushed through a circuit, work is done. The unit used to measure this work is the *watt* (abbreviated W). One watt is the work done when one volt moves one ampere:

Power = voltage × current
1 W = 1 V × 1 A

(At this time, do practice problem 6 at the end of the chapter.)

Consideration of power is important in determining whether a circuit component can withstand the amount of electricity to be passed through the circuit. The energy that a battery loses is converted to heat energy in the resistance components of a circuit. If these components are not constructed to dissipate the heat generated, the component will burn or melt. Resistors have a watt rating that must be considered when a circuit is built or repaired. For example, if a 10 kΩ resistor is rated for 2 W, can it withstand a 10 mA current?

$$W = (I) (E) = (I) (IR) = (I)^2(R)$$
$$W = (0.01 \text{ A})^2 × (10,000 \text{ Ω})$$
$$W = 0.0001 × 10,000 \text{ Ω} = 1 \text{ W}$$

Yes, 10 mA of current passing through a 10 kΩ resistance generates 1 W of energy, which can be easily dissipated by a resistor rated to dissipate twice that amount of heat.

Instruments used in the clinical laboratory are often very sophisticated and therefore expensive. In these instruments the circuits are many, complex, and intricate. With the simple insertion of a *fuse*, however, these expensive masses of electron pathways can be protected by the principle I^2R = heat.

The fuse contains a resistive element that melts at a certain temperature, causing a gap or break in the circuit. The resistive element is usually a filament of wire but can be a chemical compound, the composition of which determines its resistance and melting point. The resistance exerted by the fuse and the current through the fuse are the factors responsible for heat generation, expressed as I^2R. When sufficient heat is generated to melt the resistive element, the break in the element prevents further current conduction through the circuit. The voltage rating shown on fuses (for example, 32 V, 125 V, 250 V) indicates the size of the break or gap produced when the fuse's element melts. The larger the voltage rating, the wider the gap produced to ensure against arcing, that is, electrons jumping or a spark flying from one end of the break to the other.

The schematic symbol for a fuse is ⌒⌣. Refer to Fig. 2-7, which shows blown and good fuses. Fig. 2-8 is a representation of a circuit containing a fuse.

The line voltage (power from the wall outlet) entering an instrument is usually sent through a fuse. Therefore, if the instrument's circuit draws too much current, the fuse will prevent this excess from entering and damaging the instrument's circuitry. Other fuses may be located throughout the circuitry as protection for separate electronic circuits and/or components. Repeated blowing of fuses in an instrument is an indication that there is something electronically wrong, and the problem should be diagnosed and corrected.

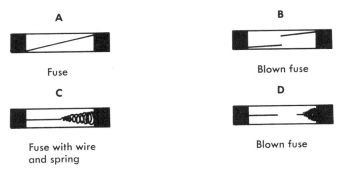

Fig. 2-7. Commonly used fuses; good fuses and blown fuses shown.

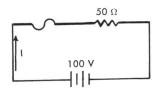

Fig. 2-8. Circuit protected with a fuse.

The fuses most commonly used in laboratory instruments are called slow-blowing fuses. These fuses do not blow immediately with a surge of current; therefore, they are said to have a high time lag. However, these fuses blow quickly if the circuit is drawing abnormally high current. These slow-blowing fuses prevent unnecessary blows resulting from high starting currents when an instrument is first turned on or from the normal surges in a commercial power supply.

Standard fuses have a short time lag; that is, they blow very quickly with increased current. This type of fuse is used to protect sensitive electronic equipment and delicate meters or components within a circuit.

ELECTRICAL GROUND

A ground is a conducting material connected to the earth. Schematically, a ground is represented as ⏚. The earth may be regarded as a "charge neutralizer." If a charged conductor is connected to the earth, the conductor will lose its charge to the earth. This conductor then will have a neutral or zero potential difference with reference to the earth or to ground.

The earth contains a tremendous accumulation of electrical charges. Therefore, it can gain or lose electrical charges while maintaining its electrical neutrality, that is, without itself becoming electrically charged. It is therefore reasonable that the ground is used as a reference point with which electrical measurements are made within a circuit. Voltage measurements at points in a circuit are taken in relationship to other points, called reference points. Frequently the reference point used is the ground or the negative side of the power source.

The chassis of an instrument may collect an electrical charge from the circuit. A connection (ground) between the metal chassis and the earth will allow the flow of the unwanted and potentially dangerous charge from the chassis to the earth. The danger in having a charge on a chassis is that an operator of that instrument may touch simultaneously the chassis and a ground (for example, a water pipe), thus becoming a conducting pathway from the chassis to earth. The resulting electrical shock is survived by the fortunate, while the less fortunate are said to have been killed by electrocution. Proper grounding is paramount in the consideration of safety.

INSTRUCTIONAL ACTIVITIES

Prior to the following exercises the instructor should demonstrate the use of a volt-ohm meter (VOM).

1. Given a VOM and six different types of material, students are to classify each type of material as an insulator or a conductor.
   Sample laboratory exercise:
   a. Distribute six types of material
      (1) Solder wire
      (2) Piece of rubber
      (3) Piece of electrical tape
      (4) Insulated wire with ends stripped
      (5) Insulated wire with ends stripped *but* wire broken and pulled slightly apart inside the insulation
      (6) Wire coated with clear nail polish
   b. Students must choose the appropriate mode of the VOM for solving the given problem.
   c. In the resistance mode of the VOM, students will observe the following meter responses with each of the given types of material:
      (1) Solder wire (low resistance) is a good conductor.
      (2) Rubber (infinite resistance) is a good insulator.
      (3) Electrical tape (infinite resistance) is a good insulator.
      (4) Insulated wire with the ends stripped (low resistance) is a good conductor.
      (5) Insulated wire with the ends stripped but the wire broken and pulled slightly apart inside the insulation will register infinite resistance in spite of the fact that metal is a good conductor. If the wire is jiggled, an intermittent response of infinite resistance-low resistance may be observed. The student should conclude that such a response could be caused by a broken wire within the insulation. This observation may be useful when troubleshooting an instrument exhibiting an abnormal intermittent signal, for example, a blinking light or an erratic meter response in a spectrophotometer.
      (6) Wire coated with clear nail polish will register infinite resistance in spite of the fact that metal is a good conductor. The student should determine the cause of this phenomenon. The student should realize the importance of metal-to-metal contact in a conducting circuit.
2. Given a VOM and two unlabelled vials, one containing distilled water and the other an electrolyte solution such as KCl, the students are to determine which solution is in each vial.
   In the resistance mode of the VOM, when the VOM's probes are inserted into the solutions, the distilled water will register a higher resistance than the electrolyte solution. This observation can be related to the use of a KCl salt bridge in electrode systems for the determination of pH, P_{CO_2}, and P_{O_2} in which KCl is a conducting medium required for completing the circuit between the reference and indicator electrodes.
3. Given a VOM and three batteries, the students are to measure the electromotive force of each battery.

4. Given a VOM and five color-coded resistors, the students are to determine the resistance of each resistor by
   a. Reading the color code on the resistor
   b. Using the VOM
   The students are then to determine whether the measured resistance is within the tolerance limits of each resistor.
5. Given a VOM, a battery, three resistors with values ranging from 1 kΩ to 5 kΩ, and wire leads with alligator clips on each end, the students are to build a circuit with the battery and the three resistors connected in series as shown below:

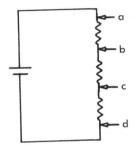

Each student should:
   a. Measure voltage at points *a*, *b*, *c*, and *d* with reference to the negative side of the battery
   b. Calculate voltage at points *a*, *b*, *c*, and *d*
   c. Explain the discrepancies between the measured and calculated values (The calculated values do not account for the internal resistance of the battery and the resistance of the connecting leads.)
6. Demonstrate the consequences of using a resistor with an inadequate power rating in a circuit. This situation may result from:
   a. A resistor of inadequate power rating being placed in a circuit during repair
   b. An increase in current because of a short or a component breakdown in a circuit

   To demonstrate, place in a circuit a resistor that has a power rating less than that required in the circuit. The resistor will be scorched by the excess heat generated. For example, if a 10 Ω (0.25 W) resistor is placed across a 3 V battery, the resistor will be scorched, since 0.9 W will be dissipated in this resistor rated for only 0.25 W.
7. Demonstrate the principle of the fuse as a protective component in a circuit. Build a circuit as shown below:

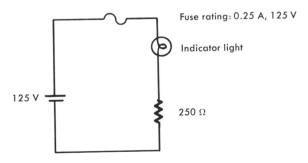

The current in the circuit is 0.5 A. The fuse will blow (the filament will melt), since it will not withstand the heat generated by the current passing through the circuit.

PRACTICE PROBLEMS and STUDY QUESTIONS

1. If 6.24×10^{18} electrons pass a point in a circuit every 10 seconds, what is the current flowing in that circuit?
2. If 3.12×10^{17} electrons pass a point in a circuit every second, what is the current flowing in that circuit?
3. A current of 100 mA is flowing in a circuit.
   a. How many electrons pass a point in the circuit every second?
   b. How many coulombs pass a point in the circuit every second?
4. If 1.56×10^{18} electrons pass through a 200 Ω resistor every 2 seconds:
   a. What is the current in this circuit?
   b. What EMF is needed to force this many electrons through the circuit at the given rate?
5. Using the following equations, derive three equations each for power, current, voltage, and resistance: $P = I \times E$ and $E = I \times R$. (In other words, express power in terms of I, E, and R; current in terms of E, R, and P; voltage in terms of I, R, and P; and resistance in term of I, E, and P.)
6. An electrical system draws 1.5 A at 100 V. How much power does the system use?
7. A 2.5 kΩ resistor is in a circuit that will carry a current of 20 mA. What is the minimum watt rating required for this resistor to be able to withstand the heat generated in this circuit?
8.

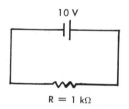

10 V

R = 1 kΩ

   a. Indicate with an arrow on the circuit diagram the direction of conventional current flow.
   b. Using + and −, indicate on the diagram the polarity of the battery.
   c. What is the current in this circuit?
   d. What amount of power does the resistor dissipate?
9.

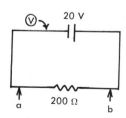

20 V

a   200 Ω   b

   a. What is the voltage at point *a* with reference to point *x*?
   b. What is the voltage at point *b* with reference to point *x*?
   c. What is the current in this circuit?
   d. What is the IR drop over the resistor?
   e. What is the voltage drop over the resistor?

10.

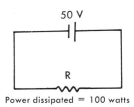

Power dissipated = 100 watts

    a. What is the current in this circuit?
    b. What is the value of R?
    c. What is the voltage drop over R?

11.

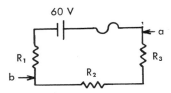

$R_1 = 1$ kΩ
$R_2 = 1$ kΩ
$R_3 = 1$ kΩ

    a. What is the current at point *b*?
    b. With reference to the battery – pole, what is the voltage· at *a*?
    c. With reference to the battery – pole, what is the voltage· at *b*?
    d. What is the minimum power rating of the fuse needed to protect this circuit?
    e. What is the current passing through this circuit?

12.

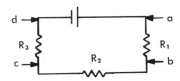

$R_1 = 200$ Ω
$R_2 = 500$ Ω
$R_3 = 300$ Ω
Power dissipated = 40 W

    a. What is the voltage of the battery?
    b. What is the current in the circuit?
    c. With reference to battery – pole, what is the voltage at *c*?
    d. With reference to battery – pole, what is the voltage at *b*?
    e. What is the current at point *c*?

13.

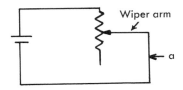

As the wiper arm on the resistor is moved in a *downward* direction in the circuit shown above, what will happen at point *a* to the voltage and to the current?

ANSWERS

1. 0.1 A or 100 mA
2. 0.05 A or 50 mA
3. a. 6.24×10^{17} electrons   b. 0.1 C
4. a. 0.125 A   b. 25 V
5. Power: $P = IE$; $P = I^2R$; $P = E^2/R$
   Current: $I = E/R$; $I = P/E$; $I = \sqrt{P/R}$
   Voltage: $E = IR$; $E = P/I$; $E = \sqrt{PR}$
   Resistance: $R = E/I$; $R = E^2/P$; $R = P/I^2$
6. 150 W
7. 1 W
8. c. 10 mA   d. 0.10 W
9. a. 0 V   b. 20 V   c. 100 mA   d. 20 V   e. 20 V
10. a. 2 A   b. 25 Ω   c. 50 V
11. a. 20 mA   b. 60 V   c. 20 V   d. 1.2 W   e. 20 mA
12. a. 200 V   b. 200 mA   c. 60 V   d. 160 V   e. 200 mA
13. Voltage is unchanged
    Current is decreased

APPROACH TO SOLVING PROBLEMS

1. 6.24×10^{18} electrons/sec = 1 A
   6.24×10^{18} electrons/10 sec = 1 A/10 = 0.1 A or 100 mA
2. $(3.12 \times 10^{17})/(6.24 \times 10^{18}$ electrons/sec) = 0.05 A or 50 mA
3. a. 0.1 A = 0.1 C
   0.1 $(6.24 \times 10^{18}$ electrons/sec) = 6.24×10^{17} electrons
   b. 0.1 C
4. a. $(1.56 \times 10^{18})/(6.24 \times 10^{18}) \times 1/2$ sec = 0.125 A
   b. $E = IR$ = 0.125 A $\times$ 200 Ω = 25 V
5. Solve by substitution in each of the two given equations.
6. $P = IE$ = 1.5 A $\times$ 100 V = 150 W
7. $P = I^2R$ = $(0.02$ A$)^2$ (2500 Ω) = (0.0004) (2500) = 1 W
8. c. $I = E/R$ = 10 V/1 kΩ = 10 mA
   d. $P = I^2R$ = $(0.01$ A$)^2 \times$ 1000 Ω = 0.10 W
9. a. Negative side of the battery is at zero potential
   b. Positive side of the battery is at potential of the battery
   c. $I = E/R$ = 20 V/200 Ω = 0.1 A
   d. All voltage is dropped over the resistor
   e. Same as (d)
10. a. $I = P/E$ = 100 W/50 V = 2 A
    b. $R = E/I$ = 50 V/2 A = 25 Ω
    c. All voltage is dropped over the resistor, 50 V
11. a. $I = E/R$ = 60 V/3 kΩ = 20 mA
    b. 60 V $\times$ 2 kΩ/3 kΩ = 40 V drop; 60 V − 40 V = 20 V
    c. Battery voltage = 60 V
    d. $P = IE$ = 0.02 A $\times$ 60 V = 1.2 W
    e. $I = E/R$ = 60 V/3 kΩ = mA
12. a. $E = \sqrt{PR} = \sqrt{(40)\,(1000)} = \sqrt{40,000}$ = 200 V
    b. $I = E/R$ = 200 V/1 kΩ = 200 mA
    c. 200 V $\times$ 700/1000 = 140 V dropped; 200 V − 140 V = 60 V
    d. 200 V $\times$ 200/1000 = 40 V dropped; 200 V − 40 V = 160 V
    e. $I = E/R$ = 200 V/1000 Ω = 200 mA or 0.2 A

CHAPTER 3

DIRECT CURRENT

Direct current is produced by batteries or by power supplies that convert alternating current to direct current. Characteristics of direct current and batteries, as a source of direct current, are described in this chapter. Instrument operators should be informed about the variety of available batteries and must be aware of the importance of required battery replacements meeting instrument specifications. Conversion of alternating current to direct current is addressed in Chapters 10 and 11 when diodes and power supplies are discussed.

CHARACTERISTICS

Direct current (dc) is characterized by the fact that both the voltage level and the polarity of the electrical charges remain unchanged over time. Current as discussed in the previous chapter was unidirectional and, therefore, direct current.

SOURCES

Sources of direct current include batteries and electronic power supplies. Most frequently, the direct current needed in circuits of clinical laboratory instruments is provided by the power supply circuit of that instrument. The power supply circuit converts alternating current to direct current by means of rectification. Material about such electronically supplied direct current will be presented when power supplies are discussed in Chapter 7.

In this chapter various types of batteries will be discussed. The purpose of presenting material about batteries is twofold—for theoretical understanding and for practical application.

1. Theoretical understanding: Parameters of voltage, potential, potential difference, and electromotive force have been defined. The various types of batteries to be discussed will demonstrate that a potential can be generated by several different chemical reactions. The common feature shared by all batteries is that positive and negative charges are developed at two different electrodes or terminals, establishing a potential difference between these terminals.

2. Practical application: Some clinical laboratory instruments do have a battery or batteries in their circuitry. These batteries are used either as a very constant dc voltage source or as a voltage reference. A battery is a component of

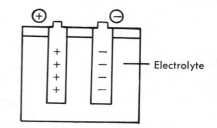

Fig. 3-1. Basic principle of battery. Potential difference between the two electrodes develops as result of chemical reaction at each.

the circuit that a laboratory scientist may be required to replace. It is therefore very important that only the type of cell required by a particular circuit is inserted into the circuit. Many batteries are similar in size, shape, color, and general appearance and may be very easily mistaken for one another. As with fuse replacement discussed earlier, battery selection is a simple but important procedure. If a battery of incorrect specifications is installed in a circuit, the circuit may be damaged or may operate inaccurately. Batteries are common everyday items. However, they usually are not given adequate consideration by laboratory personnel who should be informed about the specifications and the advantages and disadvantages of the different types. The discussion of batteries will provide the information required for understanding specific battery selection.

Basically, a battery consists of a potential difference developed as a result of a chemical reaction, as represented in Fig. 3-1. A battery is symbolically designated: ⊣|┃|┠— or simply:—⊣ ┠—. The longer vertical line represents the positive and the shorter vertical line the negative terminal of the voltage source. There are two general types of batteries, primary and secondary. The primary type of cell cannot be recharged; once it is dead, there is no resuscitation. The secondary type of cell, after being discharged, may be recharged by reversing the current through the cell. The lead-acid storage battery (car battery) is an example of a secondary cell. Since secondary cells are not used as power sources in clinical laboratory instruments, only primary cells will be discussed.

PRIMARY CELLS

The primary cells most commonly used include the carbon-zinc, the alkaline-manganese, and the zinc-mercuric oxide dry cells. A cell used not as a source of potential to force current to flow but as a reference for voltage measurement is the cadmium sulfate cell. The discussion of primary cells will include this reference cell and the other three cells mentioned.

Cadmium sulfate cell (standard Weston cell)

Accurate quantification requires that measurements be made with reference to a precisely known quantity or a standard. For the accurate measurement of voltage, a reference voltage or a standard voltage is used. Standard weights and measures are kept at the National Bureau of Standards, and so is a standard for voltage measurements. The Weston cell is almost universally used as a standard voltage.

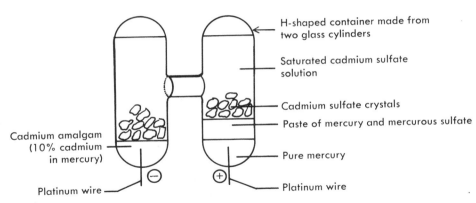

Fig. 3-2. Saturated standard Weston cell.

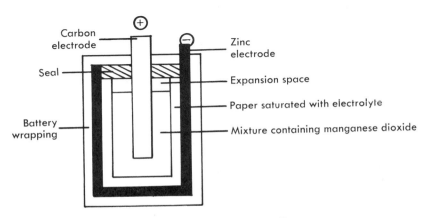

Fig. 3-3. Carbon-zinc dry cell.

The Weston reference cell can be saturated (Fig. 3-2) or unsaturated, with a potential of 1.0186 V or 1.019 V, respectively, at 20°C. The voltage decreases 4.06×10^{-5} V for each degree the temperature rises above 20°C.

Cadmium sulfate cells produce a constant voltage for many years. To provide a stable potential difference between terminals, the chemical reaction must be constant. A constant chemical reaction can be ensured only if a cell's chemical equilibrium is maintained. The equilibrium may be altered by excessive current drain or by agitation. Severe agitation can ruin a cell by causing the contents of one tube to pass through the connecting bridge and thus contaminate the contents of the other tube. In order to maintain the stability of the potential, a Weston cell is usually kept at a constant temperature and in a fixed position.

Carbon-zinc dry cell (flashlight-type battery)

An electrolyte may be absorbed by an inert material (for example, paper) or may be mixed in a paste to be used in a battery's electrochemical reaction. When such immobilized electrolyte is used in a voltage-producing cell, that cell is called a dry cell. A carbon-zinc (C-Zn) dry cell is shown in Fig. 3-3. At each of two electrodes, a chemical reaction occurs whereby the carbon electrode loses, and the zinc electrode gains, electrons. The end result is the development of a potential difference between the electrodes. A potential of 1.5 to 1.6 V is developed between the zinc *cathode,* or negative electrode, and the carbon *anode,* or positive electrode.

Thirty individual 1.5 V flashlight batteries could be connected in series (positive to negative) to produce a 45 V battery. This arrangement, however, would require too much space. Therefore, dry cell batteries are generally made by stacking alternately a carbon plate, a layer of electrolyte paste, and a zinc plate as many times as necessary to give a desired voltage. The most common dry cell batteries have voltages of 1.5, 3.0, 7.5, 22.5, 45.0, 67.5, and 90.0 V.

Batteries discharge internally when not in use. An increase in temperature increases internal discharge, thus decreasing storage life. At room temperature, the storage life of a C-Zn dry cell ranges from six months to one year.

The length of a battery's service life depends upon such factors as duration and temperature of storage before use, current drain and temperature during discharge, frequency and duration of off periods, and the quality of the battery. The service life of the C-Zn dry cell should be greater than 10 hours unless a heavy drain is placed on it. Under conditions requiring a heavy drain, frequent rest periods will extend the service life of the battery. At temperatures below freezing, this dry cell does not optimally generate a potential.

The potential of the C-Zn dry cell falls off continuously during use. The decrease in potential is caused by the change in electrolyte composition and the formation of interfering compounds during discharge. Since the potential is not constant, this battery is of little value as a reference voltage source.

The zinc casing of a C-Zn battery is the cathode (negative terminal); therefore, dissolution of zinc weakens the structure of the cell. Also, during discharge or storage, a pressure of evolved hydrogen gas builds up. This can lead to rupture of the zinc and leakage of the corrosive electrolyte into the instrument. Instruments using these dry cells should not be stored with the batteries installed.

Alkaline-manganese dry cell (alkaline cell)

The alkaline-manganese battery is similar in mechanism to the carbon-zinc dry cell but differs in electrode materials, arrangement of electrodes, and electrolyte used. The alkaline cell consists of a zinc anode, a manganese oxide cathode, and a strong alkaline electrolyte of potassium hydroxide. The alkaline cell is four times the price of the C-Zn dry cell but provides the following advantages over the C-Zn cell: the capacity (milliampere-hours) is three to five times higher; the capacity does not decrease under heavy drain; the shelf life is about two years; the internal resistance is lower, yielding higher current output; and the operating temperature limit (−40°C) is lower.

The battery is useful for applications requiring a relatively high current, which places a heavy drain on the battery. Considering its long shelf life and low operating temperature, it would be a good choice for an emergency power source.

Zinc–mercuric oxide dry cell (mercury cell)

The mercury cell generates a negative charge at the zinc amalgam anode, with the oxidation of zinc to zinc oxide yielding two electrons per atom. At the mercuric oxide – carbon cathode, a positive charge results from the reduction of mercuric oxide to mercury with the acceptance of two electrons per molecule from the carbon electrode. The resulting potential is 1.35 V, which is extremely reproducible from one cell to another. Mercury cells are available in voltages ranging from 1.35 to 42 V.

Characteristics of this dry cell include a storage life of up to two years, a service life four to five times that of the carbon-zinc dry cell, a very low internal resistance, a capacity that is greater than that of the alkaline cell but that is not maintained under heavy drain, a remarkably constant voltage during discharge, and a safe structure free of the effects of deterioration or evolved gas accumulation. The mercury cell costs about five times more than the alkaline cell, but the price is well worth the advantages gained. The high degree of voltage reproducibility between mercury cells and the virtually constant discharge voltage qualify this cell for such applications as providing potential for transistorized circuits and electrode biasing and serving as a secondary voltage standard.

The encasement of the mercury cell is less likely to leak corrosives. However, there is a slight amount of leakage that is not usually harmful to circuits. Therefore, mercury cells can be kept in instruments with relative safety. These batteries should be checked approximately every six months and any corrosive materials cleaned off.

Technologists should be aware of those instruments in which mercury cells are used (for example, the Po_2 measuring circuit frequently uses a 1.34 V mercury cell to impose a required potential across the Po_2 electrode). The voltage of this battery is constant up to the time the battery is completely discharged. This means that an instrument that is working properly may suddenly malfunction. Simple replacement of the discharged mercury cell may remedy the problem. Periodic battery replacement incorporated into a preventive maintenance schedule may prevent instrument down time resulting from battery "death." It is important not to substitute one type of battery for another. Use only the type battery specified for a particular instrument.

INSTRUCTIONAL ACTIVITIES

1. Demonstrate voltage level during current drain over a period of time for each of the following dry cells:
   a. Carbon-zinc dry cell
   b. Alkaline-manganese dry cell
   c. Zinc – mercuric oxide dry cell

   Connect each of the three dry cells in circuits with a high current drain of about 1 A. Monitor with a VOM the voltage of each cell during the period of heavy current drain.

   From the observed data, require students to draw conclusions about each of the three cells.

PRACTICE PROBLEMS and STUDY QUESTIONS

1. What is the voltage of a saturated Weston cell at 25°C?
2. List applications appropriate for each of the following electrochemical cells:
   a. Cadmium sulfate cell
   b. Carbon-zinc dry cell
   c. Alkaline-manganese dry cell
   d. Zinc–mercuric oxide dry cell
3. Matching (*Note:* Use each lettered answer at least once; some answers are to be used more than once.)

   ____ (1) Dry cell that operates at −40°C   A. Cadmium sulfate cell
   ____ (2) Dry cell with constant voltage   B. Alkaline cell
             over lifetime of cell   C. Mercury cell
   ____ (3) Standard Weston cell   D. C-Zn cell
   ____ (4) Alkaline-manganese dry cell
   ____ (5) 1.0186 V at 20°C
   ____ (6) Capacity does not fall off
             with heavy drain
   ____ (7) Zinc–mercuric oxide dry cell
   ____ (8) Dry cell with least stable voltage

ANSWERS
1. 1.0184 V
2. a. Voltage reference
   b. Inexpensive voltage source when constant voltage not required (for example, flashlight and battery-operated gadgets)
   c. Emergency power source since functional at subzero temperatures and has long shelf life
   d. Voltage source when constant voltage is required (for example, as secondary voltage standard, in transistorized circuits, and for applied voltage across an electrode)
3. (1) B
   (2) C
   (3) A
   (4) B
   (5) A
   (6) B
   (7) C
   (8) D

APPROACH TO SOLVING PROBLEMS
1. $5°C \times (4.06 \times 10^{-5} V/°C) = 2.03 \times 10^{-4} V$
   $1.0186 V$ (at 20°C) $- (0.0002) = 1.0184 V$ at 25°C

CHAPTER 4

ALTERNATING CURRENT

Alternating current is generated commercially and supplied to consumers via wall outlets. Our concern with alternating current begins when it enters electrically powered instruments. The discussion of alternating current will include its description, its relationship to direct current, and its behavior in different electronic components. This presentation will concentrate on the descriptive aspects of alternating current. The effects of different components on alternating current will be included in the discussions of the particular components. Characteristics of alternating current (ac) include constant changing of direction of current flow, voltage variation over time, amplitude, frequency, and phase. The symbolic representation of an alternating current potential source is: ─◯─ .

DIRECTION OF ALTERNATING CURRENT FLOW

Alternating current flows first in one direction and then in the opposite direction. For a more graphic description, consider the analogy of a two-lane road as a conductor and the cars as moving charges. Consider the situation in which one of the two lanes is closed. Flagmen regulate traffic flow by allowing cars (charges) to move, first in one direction and then in the other, through the constricted roadway (conductor). Thus the direction of traffic is constantly changing. Alternating current works in the same way.

VOLTAGE VARIATION OVER TIME

There are different waveforms, of which the sinusoidal waveform (Fig. 4-1) is the most common and to which this discussion will be limited. The sine wave shown in Fig. 4-1 starts at 0 V, increases over time to 10 V, then decreases to 0 V. From 0 V the polarity is reversed, and the voltage goes to −10 V, then returns to 0 V again. This is considered one complete cycle of the waveform.

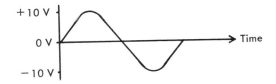

Fig. 4-1. Sinusoidal waveform.

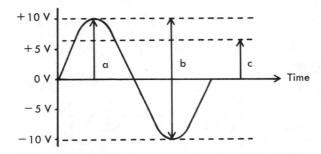

Fig. 4-2. AC voltage; a = peak amplitude or peak voltage; b = peak-to-peak amplitude or peak-to-peak voltage; c = root mean square (rms) value of voltage (rms = peak voltage [× 0.707]).

AMPLITUDE

The amplitude of the waveform is the peak value of the voltage. Refer to Fig. 4-2. Peak-to-peak amplitude or voltage is the total voltage in both directions from 0 V. For example, in Fig. 4-2 the voltage reads 10 V in one direction and 10 V in the other direction. Therefore, the total voltage, or peak-to-peak voltage, is 20 V. Peak voltage is voltage in one direction only (for example, 10 V in Fig. 4-2).

In the discussion of voltage, it would be convenient to be able to equate dc voltage with ac voltage. As a matter of fact, volt-ohm meters do read ac voltage in values equivalent to dc voltage. This equivalent dc voltage, which may be considered an average of ac voltage, is less than peak voltage by a factor of 0.707. That is:

ac peak voltage × 0.707 = root-mean-square (rms) voltage

The rms value of ac voltage is comparable to dc voltage in considering the amount of heat generated by ac and dc. To convert rms value to peak value:

rms × 1.41 = peak value

For example, if a voltage from a wall outlet of 110 volts ac (Vac) is the rms value, what is the peak value?

Peak value = rms value × 1.41
Peak value = 110 V × 1.41 = 155.1 Vac

FREQUENCY

One complete waveform is one cycle. The number of cycles occurring each second is the frequency of the waveform. The commercially supplied ac in the United States has a frequency of 60 cycles per second (c/s), or using the preferred terminology, 60 hertz (Hz). In other countries ac current is generated at a frequency of 50 Hz.

The time required for one cycle is a period. The relationship of the period (T) and the frequency (F) of a signal is reciprocal:

Period = 1/frequency or T = 1/F
Frequency = 1/period or F = 1/T

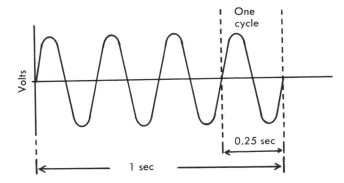

Fig. 4-3. Frequency and period of waveform; frequency (F) = 4 cycles per second (c/s) or hertz (Hz); period (T) = time required for 1 cycle = 0.25 second; equations: F = 1/T and T = 1/F.

Refer to Fig. 4-3. One cycle occurs every 0.25 sec; therefore, the period is 0.25 sec. The frequency is 4 Hz, since four cycles occur every second. Calculate these values:

F = 1/T = 1/0.25 sec = 4 Hz
T = 1/F = 1/4 Hz = 0.25 sec

Note: Audio frequency range = 20 Hz to 20,000 Hz
Radio frequency range = 100 kHz to 30 MHz

PHASE

Using one signal as a reference, a time relationship (a phase difference) can be determined between that signal and another signal or signals.

Fig. 4-4, *A*, shows the periodic plotting of a waveform. Fig. 4-4, *B*, shows two waveforms or signals in phase. When signal 1 is at its maximum positive swing, so is signal 2, and when signal 1 is at its maximum negative swing, so is signal 2. If these two signals were added together, the resultant signal would have an amplitude equal to the sum of the amplitudes of signals 1 and 2. That is:

Amplitude of signal 1 + amplitude of signal 2 = amplitude of resultant signal 3

Fig. 4-4, *C*, represents two signals that are out of phase. If two such voltages, both of equal magnitude, were introduced into a circuit, the resultant voltage felt by the circuit would be 0 V, since one signal cancels the other.

INSTRUCTIONAL ACTIVITIES

1. Using an oscilloscope and an audio-signal generator, demonstrate the characteristics of the following electrical signals:
   a. Direct current
      (1) Unidirectional
      (2) Amplitude unchanged over time
   b. Alternating current — sine waveform
      (1) Alternating direction change in current flow
      (2) Voltage variation over time
      (3) Peak-to-peak voltage
      (4) Root-mean-square voltage

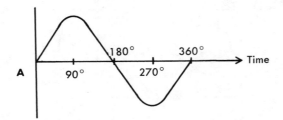

Relative degrees in ac sinewave

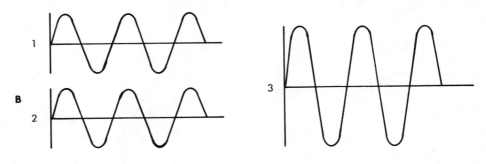

Signals 1 and 2 180° out of phase added to give signal 3

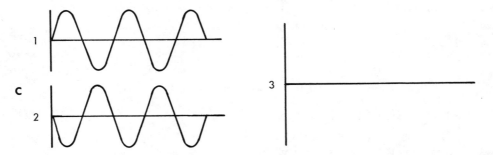

Signals 1 and 2 added to give signal 3

Fig. 4-4. Periodic plotting of sinewave.

(5) Frequency

(6) Period

(7) Phase

2. Demonstrate "the sights and sounds of electricity." Connect to an audio-signal generator an oscilloscope and an inexpensive speaker.

a. Change the frequency of the signal from 20 Hz to 20,000 Hz. The frequency change can be seen on the oscilloscope and can be heard through the speaker. A low pitched tone is heard around 20 Hz. The tone becomes higher pitched as the frequency is increased, and a very high pitched tone disappears around 20,000 Hz. This illustrates that the audio range extends from 20 Hz to 20,000 Hz. Two sensory perceptions of frequency change provide a strong impression of the meaning of frequency.

b. With the audio-signal generator set at a frequency comfortable to listen to (for example, 10,000 Hz), change the voltage and thus the amplitude of the signal. With increased voltage the waveform's amplitude increases. This is seen on the oscilloscope and heard through the speaker as an increase in volume. The opposite is true of a decrease in voltage. Here again, two sensory perceptions of voltage change provide a strong impression of the meaning of amplitude.

PRACTICE PROBLEMS and STUDY QUESTIONS

1.

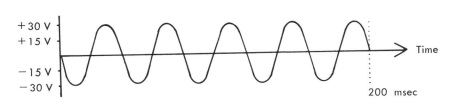

a. Is the above signal ac or dc?

b. What is the waveform of the above signal?

c. What are the following values for the waveform shown?

(1) Amplitude

(2) Peak-to-peak voltage

(3) Peak voltage

(4) Root-mean-square voltage

(5) Frequency

(6) Period

2.

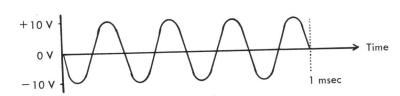

What are the following values for the waveform shown above?

a. Amplitude

b. Peak-to-peak voltage

c. Peak voltage

d. Root-mean-square voltage

e. Frequency

f. Period

3. What are the peak amplitudes of signals having the following rms values?
   a. 100 V
   b. 75 V
   c. 115 V
   d. 50 V

4.

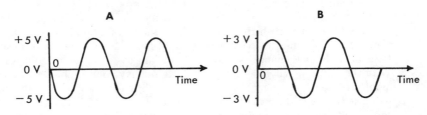

a. How many degrees out of phase are waveforms A and B?
b. If these two waveforms were added together, what would the peak-to-peak amplitude of the resultant waveform be?

ANSWERS

1. a. ac
   b. Sine waveform
   c. (1) 30 V
      (2) 60 V
      (3) 30 V
      (4) 21.21 V
      (5) 25 Hz
      (6) 0.04 sec

2. a. 10 V
   b. 20 V
   c. 10 V
   d. 7.07 V
   e. 4000 Hz
   f. 0.25 msec

3. a. 141 V
   b. 105.75 V
   c. 162.15 V
   d. 70.5 V

4. a. 180°
   b. 4 V

APPROACH TO SOLVING PROBLEMS

1. c. (1) Maximum voltage in one direction is 30 V
      (2) 30 V + 30 V = 60 V
      (3) Same as amplitude
      (4) rms = 0.707 × peak = 0.707 × 30 V = 21.21 V
      (5) 5 cycles/200 msec or 25 c/s = 25 Hz
      (6) P = 1/F = 1/25 = 0.04 sec

2. a. Maximum voltage in one direction is 10 V
   b. 10 V + 10 V = 20 V
   c. Same as amplitude
   d. 10 V × 0.707 = 7.07 V
   e. 4 cycles/msec = 4000 c/s = 4000 Hz
   f. P = 1/F = 1/4000 = 0.25 msec

3. a. Peak value = rms × 1.41 = 100 V × 1.41 = 141 V
   b. Peak value = rms × 1.41 = 75 V × 1.41 = 105.75 V
   c. Peak value = rms × 1.41 = 115 V × 1.41 = 162.15 V
   d. Peak value = rms × 1.41 = 50 V × 1.41 = 70.5 V

4. b. Addition of these two waveforms results in a waveform with a peak value of 2 V; therefore, the peak-to-peak value is:
      2 V + 2 V = 4 V.

Electronic components

Electronic circuits consist of a variety of electronic components specifically selected and purposefully arranged so as to perform particular operations. Of the commonly used components, those to be discussed in this section are resistors, capacitors, inductors, transformers, and diodes. Discussion of each component will include construction, function, effect on alternating and direct current, and representative electronic symbols. The collection of isolated facts and figures in this section will be used in Section Four to illustrate the interrelatedness of component functions in analytical instruments' functional units, for example, power supply.

CHAPTER 5

CIRCUIT CONFIGURATIONS

Circuit configuration is the arrangement of electronic components in a circuit. Components may be connected in series, in parallel, or in a combination of series and parallel. In this chapter different circuit configurations will be illustrated by using that familiar component, the resistor.

Two commonly used methods of representing connections in an electrical circuit are shown in Fig. 5-1, *A* and *B*. Circuits may be drawn so that a node or dot at the point of intersection of lines represents an electrical connection as shown in Fig. 5-1, *A*. In this circuit representation the intersections at points *a* and *b* are not making electrical contact. In Fig. 5-1, *B*, intersecting straight lines represent electrical contact points, while the arched lines at points *a* and *b* indicate that these are not electrical connections. This latter type of circuit representation is used in the illustrations throughout this text.

SERIES CIRCUIT

Refer to Fig. 5-2, in which three resistors are connected in series in a circuit. A component is connected in series when it is connected to other components in such a way that current flow has only one possible pathway.

The total resistance exerted by resistors in series is calculated thus:

$$R_{total} = R_1 + R_2 + R_3 + R_4 + \ldots R_n$$

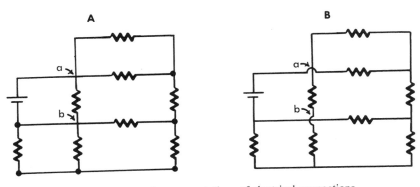

Fig. 5-1. Schematic representations of electrical connections.

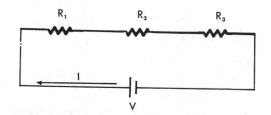

Fig. 5-2. Series combination of resistors.

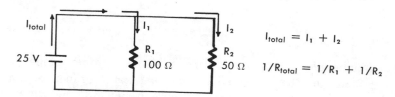

Fig. 5-3. Parallel circuit.

PARALLEL CIRCUITS

Fig. 5-3 shows two resistors connected in parallel. The same voltage is dropped across each resistor. However, the current flow has two alternate paths to follow. When current has a choice of pathways, the conducting pathways are connected in parallel.

The total current in a circuit is equal to the sum of the current in all parallel pathways in the circuit. The total current in the circuit shown in Fig. 5-3 is equal to the sum of the current passing through R_1 and R_2:

$$I_{total} = I_1 + I_2$$

What are the values for I_1 and I_2?

$$I_1 = V/R_1 = 25 \text{ V}/100 \ \Omega = 0.25 \text{ A}$$

$$I_2 = V/R_2 = 25 \text{ V}/50 \ \Omega = 0.50 \text{ A}$$

What is the total current in this circuit?

$$I_{total} = I_1 + I_2 = 0.25 \text{ A} + 0.50 \text{ A} = 0.75 \text{ A}$$

The resistance to current flow in this circuit is less than if these resistors were connected in series. When resistors are connected in series, the voltage from the voltage source is dropped across all of them. That is, the voltage source "sees" an "effective" resistance equal to the sum of the resistors in series. However, when the resistors are in parallel, the full voltage is dropped across each resistor separately. A current flows in each resistor independently of the current in the other resistors in the parallel circuit. The total effective resistance in a parallel circuit is always less than the smallest resistor. The formula for calculating the total effective resistance in a parallel circuit is:

$$1/R_{total} = 1/R_1 + 1/R_2 + 1/R_3 + \ldots 1/R_n$$

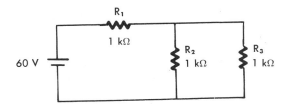

Fig. 5-4. Series-parallel circuit.

Referring to the circuit in Fig. 5-3, note the following example. What is the total "effective" resistance in this circuit?

$$1/R_{total} = 1/R_1 + 1/R_2$$
$$1/R_{total} = (R_1 + R_2)/(R_1R_2)$$
$$R_{total} = (R_1R_2)/(R_1 + R_2)$$
$$R_{total} = [(100\ \Omega)\ (50\ \Omega)]/(100\ \Omega + 50\ \Omega) = 5000\ \Omega/150\ \Omega = 33.33\ \Omega$$

If the 100 Ω and 50 Ω resistors were replaced with a 33.33 Ω resistor, what current would flow in this circuit?

$$I = E/R = 25\ V/33.33\ \Omega = 0.75\ A$$

Note that calculating total current in this circuit by adding the current flowing through each resistor results in the same value of 0.75 A.

SERIES-PARALLEL CIRCUITS

Series circuits and parallel circuits have been discussed. A third possible variation of circuit design is a combination series-parallel circuit as shown in Fig. 5-4.

If the effective resistance of R_2 and R_3 is calculated, the two parallel limbs are essentially changed to a series with R_1. The effective resistance of R_2 and R_3 is:

$$1/R_{total} = 1/R_2 + 1/R_3$$
$$1/R_{total} = 1/1000\ \Omega + 1/1000\ \Omega = 2/1000\ \Omega = 1/500\ \Omega$$
$$R_{total} = 500\ \Omega$$

The total effective resistance of the entire circuit then becomes:

$$R = R_1 + \text{(effective resistance of } R_2 \text{ and } R_3)$$
$$R = 1000\ \Omega + 500\ \Omega$$
$$R = 1500\ \Omega$$

Current flow in this system is more complex than in either a series or a parallel circuit. The entire current of the circuit must flow through R_1. This same current then will find two paths, R_2 and R_3, between which it will be divided.

Current flow in the entire system is calculated by using the total resistance of 1500 Ω.

$$I = E/R = 60\ V/1500\ \Omega = 40\ mA$$

Notice that the sum of the current in the parallel limbs is the same as that flowing through the series portion of the circuit, which must carry the total current. Using the above approach, a complex series-parallel combination of resistors can be analyzed and the effective resistance of the circuit calculated.

Voltage drop, voltage division, and current division are important electronic concepts that must be understood. Comprehension of these concepts will provide a strong foundation upon which other theories and concepts can be built. Therefore, it is strongly recommended that the instructional unit "Voltage Division and Current Division" (pp. 51 to 56) be studied and that all the practice problems be worked.

INSTRUCTIONAL ACTIVITIES

1. Have students work through the instructional unit on voltage division and current division at the end of this chapter.
2. Demonstrate an approach to calculating designated values in the series-parallel circuit as shown in the following illustration.

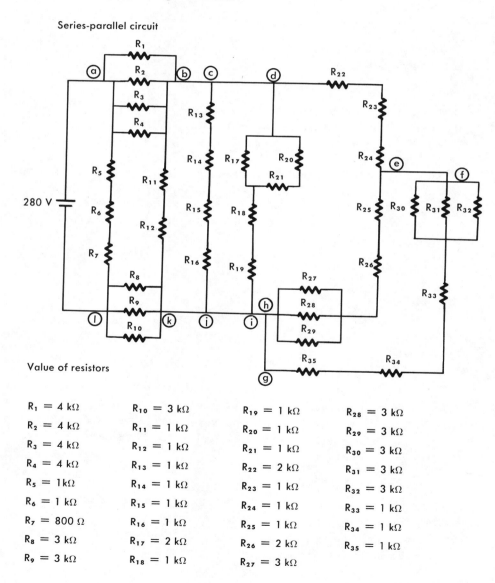

Series-parallel circuit

Value of resistors

$R_1 = 4\ k\Omega$	$R_{10} = 3\ k\Omega$	$R_{19} = 1\ k\Omega$	$R_{28} = 3\ k\Omega$
$R_2 = 4\ k\Omega$	$R_{11} = 1\ k\Omega$	$R_{20} = 1\ k\Omega$	$R_{29} = 3\ k\Omega$
$R_3 = 4\ k\Omega$	$R_{12} = 1\ k\Omega$	$R_{21} = 1\ k\Omega$	$R_{30} = 3\ k\Omega$
$R_4 = 4\ k\Omega$	$R_{13} = 1\ k\Omega$	$R_{22} = 2\ k\Omega$	$R_{31} = 3\ k\Omega$
$R_5 = 1 k\Omega$	$R_{14} = 1\ k\Omega$	$R_{23} = 1\ k\Omega$	$R_{32} = 3\ k\Omega$
$R_6 = 1\ k\Omega$	$R_{15} = 1\ k\Omega$	$R_{24} = 1\ k\Omega$	$R_{33} = 1\ k\Omega$
$R_7 = 800\ \Omega$	$R_{16} = 1\ k\Omega$	$R_{25} = 1\ k\Omega$	$R_{34} = 1\ k\Omega$
$R_8 = 3\ k\Omega$	$R_{17} = 2\ k\Omega$	$R_{26} = 2\ k\Omega$	$R_{35} = 1\ k\Omega$
$R_9 = 3\ k\Omega$	$R_{18} = 1\ k\Omega$	$R_{27} = 3\ k\Omega$	

Calculate:
a. Total effective resistance
b. Total current
c. Total power dissipated
d. Voltage drop over each resistor
e. Current through each resistor

a. Total effective resistance = 1.4 kΩ = total R$_{eff}$. The effective resistances calculated on p. 44 are used as resistance values in the equivalent circuits in the following illustration.

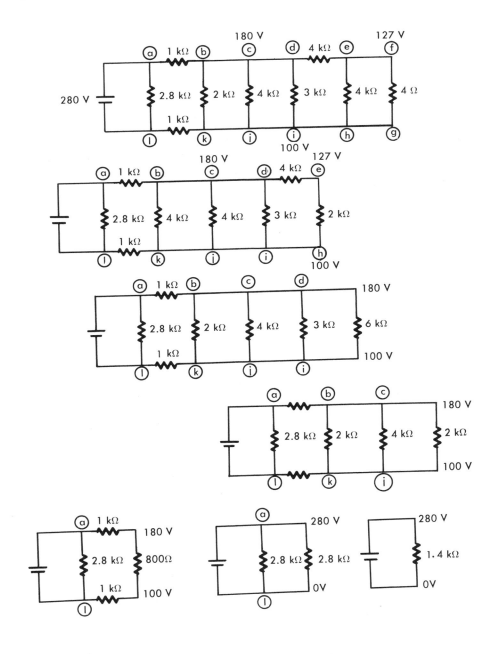

$$1/R_{total} = 1/R_1 + 1/R_2 + 1/R_3 + 1/R_4 = 4/4 \text{ k}\Omega : R_{total} = 1 \text{ k}\Omega$$
$$1/R_{total} = 1/R_8 + 1/R_9 + 1/R_{10} = 3/3 \text{ k}\Omega : R_{total} = 1 \text{ k}\Omega$$
$$R_{total} = R_5 + R_6 + R_7 = 1 \text{ k}\Omega + 1 \text{ k}\Omega + 800 \text{ }\Omega = 2.8 \text{ k}\Omega$$
$$R_{total} = R_{11} + R_{12} = 1 \text{ k}\Omega + 1 \text{ k}\Omega = 2 \text{ k}\Omega$$
$$R_{total} = R_{13} + R_{14} + R_{15} + R_{16} = 1 \text{ k}\Omega + 1 \text{ k}\Omega + 1 \text{ k}\Omega + 1 \text{ k}\Omega = 4 \text{ k}\Omega$$
$$1/R_{total} = 1/R_{17} + [1/(R_{20} + R_{21})] = 1/2 \text{ k}\Omega + 1/2 \text{ k}\Omega = 1 \text{ k}\Omega : R_{total} = 1 \text{ k}\Omega$$
$$R_{total} = R_{18} + R_{19} = 2 \text{ k}\Omega$$
$$R_{total} = R_{22} + R_{23} + R_{24} = 4 \text{ k}\Omega$$
$$1/R_{total} = 1/R_{30} + 1/R_{31} + 1/R_{32} = 1 \text{ k}\Omega : R_{total} = 1 \text{ k}\Omega$$
$$R_{total} = R_{25} + R_{26} = 3 \text{ k}\Omega$$
$$1/R_{total} = 1/R_{27} + 1/R_{28} + 1/R_{29} = 1 \text{ k}\Omega : R_{total} = 1 \text{ k}\Omega$$
$$R_{total} = R_{33} + R_{34} + R_{35} = 3 \text{ k}\Omega$$

b. Total current: $I_{total} = V/R_{eff} = 280 \text{ V}/1.4 \text{ k}\Omega = 200 \text{ mA}$

c. Total power dissipated: $P = I \; E = (0.2 \text{ A}) (280 \text{ V}) = 56$ watts

d. Voltage drop over each resistor:

R_1: 100 V	R_{10}: 100 V	R_{19}: 26.7 V	R_{28}: 6.8 V
R_2: 100 V	R_{11}: 40 V	R_{20}: 13.4 V	R_{29}: 6.8 V
R_3: 100 V	R_{12}: 40 V	R_{21}: 13.4 V	R_{30}: 6.8 V
R_4: 100 V	R_{13}: 20 V	R_{22}: 26.5 V	R_{31}: 6.8 V
R_5: 100 V	R_{14}: 20 V	R_{23}: 13.3 V	R_{32}: 6.8 V
R_6: 100 V	R_{15}: 20 V	R_{24}: 13.3 V	R_{33}: 6.8 V
R_7: 80 V	R_{16}: 20 V	R_{25}: 6.8 V	R_{34}: 6.8 V
R_8: 100 V	R_{17}: 26.7 V	R_{26}: 13.5 V	R_{35}: 6.8 V
R_9: 100 V	R_{18}: 26.7 V	R_{27}: 6.8 V	

e. Current through each resistor:

R_1: 25 mA	R_{10}: 33.3 mA	R_{19}: 26.7 mA	R_{28}: 2.3 mA
R_2: 25 mA	R_{11}: 40 mA	R_{20}: 13.4 mA	R_{29}: 2.3 mA
R_3: 25 mA	R_{12}: 40 mA	R_{21}: 13.4 mA	R_{30}: 2.3 mA
R_4: 25 mA	R_{13}: 20 mA	R_{22}: 13.3 mA	R_{31}: 2.3 mA
R_5: 100 mA	R_{14}: 20 mA	R_{23}: 13.3 mA	R_{32}: 2.3 mA
R_6: 100 mA	R_{15}: 20 mA	R_{24}: 13.3 mA	R_{33}: 6.8 mA
R_7: 125 mA	R_{16}: 20 mA	R_{25}: 6.8 mA	R_{34}: 6.8 mA
R_8: 33.3 mA	R_{17}: 13.35 mA	R_{26}: 6.8 mA	R_{35}: 6.8 mA
R_9: 33.3 mA	R_{18}: 26.7 mA	R_{27}: 2.3 mA	

PRACTICE PROBLEMS and STUDY QUESTIONS

1. For each of the following circuits calculate:
   a. Total effective resistance
   b. Current drawn from the battery
   c. Voltage drop over each resistor
   d. Current passing through each resistor
   e. Voltage at points a, b, c, and d
   f. Power dissipated

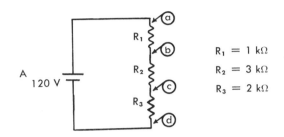

$R_1 = 1\ k\Omega$
$R_2 = 3\ k\Omega$
$R_3 = 2\ k\Omega$

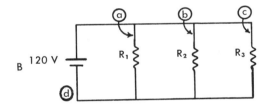

$R_1 = 1\ k\Omega$
$R_2 = 3\ k\Omega$
$R_3 = 2\ k\Omega$

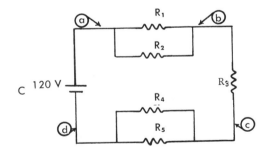

$R_1 = 6\ k\Omega$
$R_2 = 2\ k\Omega$
$R_3 = 2\ k\Omega$
$R_4 = 3\ k\Omega$
$R_5 = 3\ k\Omega$

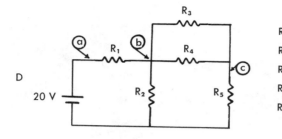

$R_1 = 1 \text{ k}\Omega$
$R_2 = 2 \text{ k}\Omega$
$R_3 = 2 \text{ k}\Omega$
$R_4 = 2 \text{ k}\Omega$
$R_5 = 1 \text{ k}\Omega$

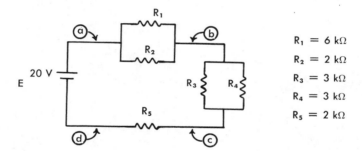

$R_1 = 6 \text{ k}\Omega$
$R_2 = 2 \text{ k}\Omega$
$R_3 = 3 \text{ k}\Omega$
$R_4 = 3 \text{ k}\Omega$
$R_5 = 2 \text{ k}\Omega$

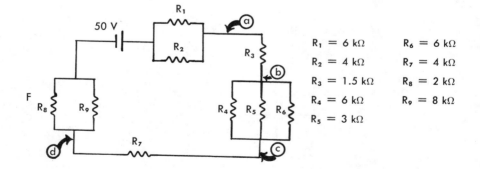

$R_1 = 6 \text{ k}\Omega$ $R_6 = 6 \text{ k}\Omega$
$R_2 = 4 \text{ k}\Omega$ $R_7 = 4 \text{ k}\Omega$
$R_3 = 1.5 \text{ k}\Omega$ $R_8 = 2 \text{ k}\Omega$
$R_4 = 6 \text{ k}\Omega$ $R_9 = 8 \text{ k}\Omega$
$R_5 = 3 \text{ k}\Omega$

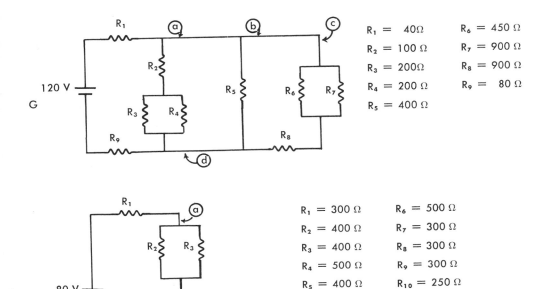

R₁ = 40Ω   R₆ = 450 Ω
R₂ = 100 Ω   R₇ = 900 Ω
R₃ = 200Ω   R₈ = 900 Ω
R₄ = 200 Ω   R₉ = 80 Ω
R₅ = 400 Ω

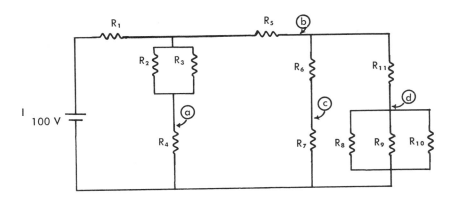

R₁ = 300 Ω   R₆ = 500 Ω
R₂ = 400 Ω   R₇ = 300 Ω
R₃ = 400 Ω   R₈ = 300 Ω
R₄ = 500 Ω   R₉ = 300 Ω
R₅ = 400 Ω   R₁₀ = 250 Ω

R₁ = 5 kΩ
R₂ = 10 kΩ
R₃ = 10 kΩ
R₄ = 5 kΩ
R₅ = 5 kΩ
R₆ = 5 kΩ
R₇ = 5 kΩ
R₈ = 15 kΩ
R₉ = 15 kΩ
R₁₀ = 15 kΩ
R₁₁ = 5 kΩ

2. For the following circuit calculate:
   a. Voltage drop over each branch, 1, 2, and 3
   b. Voltage drop over each resistor
   c. Current drawn from the battery
   d. Current flowing in each branch, 1, 2, and 3
   e. Current through each resistor
   Note: Analyze your results, and review the concepts of voltage division and current division as demonstrated in this circuit.

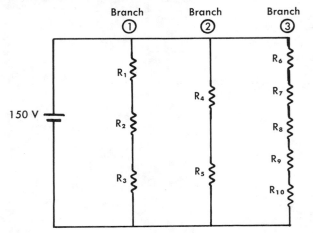

$$R_1 = 1 \text{ k}\Omega$$
$$R_2 = 1 \text{ k}\Omega$$
$$R_3 = 1 \text{ k}\Omega$$
$$R_4 = 250 \ \Omega$$
$$R_5 = 750 \ \Omega$$
$$R_6 = 100 \ \Omega$$
$$R_7 = 300 \ \Omega$$
$$R_8 = 200 \ \Omega$$
$$R_9 = 50 \ \Omega$$
$$R_{10} = 350 \ \Omega$$

3. For the following circuit calculate:
   a. Total effective resistance
   b. Current drawn from the battery
   c. Total current in the circuit (I_{total})
   d. The power dissipated in the circuit
   e. Voltage drop over each resistor
   f. Current through each resistor
   g. Currents I_1, I_2, and I_3

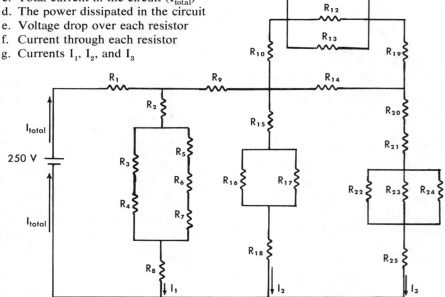

$$R_1 = 1083 \ \Omega$$

All other resistors = 1 kΩ

ANSWERS

1. Fig. *A* a. 6 kΩ   c. R₁: 20 V   d. R₁: 20 mA   e. a: 120 V   f. 2.4 W
            b. 20 mA   R₂: 60 V   R₂: 20 mA   b: 100 V
                         R₃: 40 V   R₃: 20 mA   c: 40 V
                                                           d: 0 V

   Fig. *B* a. 545 Ω   c. R₁: 120 V   d. R₁: 120 mA   e. a: 120 V   f. 26.4 W
            b. 220 mA   R₂: 120 V   R₂: 40 mA   b: 120 V
                         R₃: 120 V   R₃: 60 mA   c: 120 V
                                                           d: 0 V

   Fig. *C* a. 5 kΩ   c. R₁: 36 V   d. R₁: 6 mA   e. a: 120 V   f. 2.88 W
            b. 24 mA   R₂: 36 V   R₂: 18 mA   b: 84 V
                         R₃: 48 V   R₃: 24 mA   c: 36 V
                         R₄: 36 V   R₄: 12 mA   d: 0 V
                         R₅: 36 V   R₅: 12 mA

   Fig. *D* a. 2 kΩ   c. R₁: 10 V   d. R₁: 10 mA   e. a: 20 V   f. 0.2 W
            b. 10 mA   R₂: 10 V   R₂: 5 mA   b: 10 V
                         R₃: 5 V   R₃: 2.5 mA   c: 5 V
                         R₄: 5 V   R₄: 2.5 mA   d: 0 V
                         R₅: 5 V   R₅: 5 mA

   Fig. *E* a. 5 kΩ   c. R₁: 6 V   d. R₁: 1 mA   e. a: 20 V   f. 0.08 W
            b. 4 mA   R₂: 6 V   R₂: 3 mA   b: 14 V
                         R₃: 6 V   R₃: 2 mA   c: 8 V
                         R₄: 6 V   R₄: 2 mA   d: 0 V
                         R₅: 8 V   R₅: 4 mA

   Fig. *F* a. 11 kΩ   c. R₁: 10.9 V   d. R₁: 1.82 mA e. a: 39.1 V   f. 0.227 W
            b. 4.545 mA R₂: 10.9 V   R₂: 2.72 mA   b: 32.3 V
                         R₃: 6.8 V   R₃: 4.53 mA   c: 25.5 V
                         R₄: 6.8 V   R₄: 1.13 mA   d: 7.3 V
                         R₅: 6.8 V   R₅: 2.26 mA
                         R₆: 6.8 V   R₆: 1.13 mA
                         R₇: 18.2 V   R₇: 4.55 mA
                         R₈: 7.3 V   R₈: 3.65 mA
                         R₉: 7.3 V   R₉: 0.91 mA

   Fig. *G* a. 240 Ω   c. R₁: 20 V   d. R₁: 0.5 A   e. a: 100 V   f. 60 W
            b. 0.5 A   R₂: 30 V   R₂: 0.3 A   b: 100 V
                         R₃: 30 V   R₃: 0.15 A   c: 100 V
                         R₄: 30 V   R₄: 0.15 A   d: 40 V
                         R₅: 60 V   R₅: 0.15 A
                         R₆: 15 V   R₆: 0.033 A
                         R₇: 15 V   R₇: 0.016 A
                         R₈: 45 V   R₈: 0.05 A
                         R₉: 40 V   R₉: 0.5 A

   Fig. *H* a. 1.6 kΩ   c. R₁: 15 V   d. R₁: 50 mA   e. a: 65 V   f. 4 W
            b. 50 mA   R₂: 10 V   R₂: 25 mA   b: 25 V
                         R₃: 10 V   R₃: 25 mA   c: 15 V
                         R₄: 30 V   R₄: 50 mA   d: 12.5 V
                         R₅: 10 V   R₅: 25 mA
                         R₆: 12.5 V   R₆: 25 mA
                         R₇: 2.5 V   R₇: 8.3 mA
                         R₈: 2.5 V   R₈: 8.3 mA
                         R₉: 2.5 V   R₉: 8.3 mA
                         R₁₀: 12.5 V   R₁₀: 50 mA

Fig. *I* a. 10 kΩ
  b. 10 mA

c. R_1: 50 V
  R_2: 25 V
  R_3: 25 V
  R_4: 25 V
  R_5: 25 V
  R_6: 12.5 V
  R_7: 12.5 V
  R_8: 12.5 V
  R_9: 12.5 V
  R_{10}: 12.5 V
  R_{11}: 12.5 V

d. R_1: 10 mA
  R_2: 2.5 mA
  R_3: 2.5 mA
  R_4: 5 mA
  R_5: 5 mA
  R_6: 2.5 mA
  R_7: 2.5 mA
  R_8: 0.83 mA
  R_9: 0.83 mA
  R_{10}: 0.83 mA
  R_{11}: 2.5 mA

e. a: 25 V
  b: 25 V
  c: 12.5 V
  d: 12.5 V

f. 1 W

2. a. branch 1: 150 V
  branch 2: 150 V
  branch 3: 150 V

b. R_1: 50 V
  R_2: 50 V
  R_3: 50 V
  R_4: 37.5 V
  R_5: 112.5 V
  R_6: 15.0 V
  R_7: 45.0 V
  R_8: 30.0 V
  R_9: 7.5 V
  R_{10}: 52.5 V

c. 350 mA
d. branch 1: 50 mA
  branch 2: 150 mA
  branch 3: 150 mA

e. R_1: 50 mA
  R_2: 50 mA
  R_3: 50 mA
  R_4: 150 mA
  R_5: 150 mA
  R_6: 150 mA
  R_7: 150 mA
  R_8: 150 mA
  R_9: 150 mA
  R_{10}: 150 mA

3. a. 2.5 kΩ
  b. 100 mA
  c. 100 mA
  d. 25 W

e. R_1: 108.3 V
  R_2: 44.28 V
  R_3: 26.57 V
  R_4 26.57 V
  R_5: 17.71 V
  R_6: 17.71 V
  R_7: 17.71 V
  R_8: 44.28 V
  R_9: 55.72 V
  R_{10}: 6.4 V
  R_{11}: 2.13 V
  R_{12}: 2.13 V
  R_{13}: 2.13 V
  R_{14}: 14.92 V
  R_{15}: 34.39 V
  R_{16}: 17.2 V
  R_{17}: 17.2 V
  R_{18}: 34.39 V
  R_{19}: 6.4 V
  R_{20}: 21.32 V
  R_{21}: 21.32 V
  R_{22}: 7.11 V
  R_{23}: 7.11 V
  R_{24}: 7.11 V
  R_{25}: 21.32 V

f. R_1: 100 mA
  R_2: 44.28 mA
  R_3: 26.57 mA
  R_4: 26.57 mA
  R_5: 17.71 mA
  R_6: 17.71 mA
  R_7: 17.71 mA
  R_8: 44.28 mA
  R_9: 55.72 mA
  R_{10}: 6.4 mA
  R_{11}: 2.13 mA
  R_{12}: 2.13 mA
  R_{13}: 2.13 mA
  R_{14}: 14.92 mA
  R_{15}: 34.39 mA
  R_{16}: 17.2 mA
  R_{17}: 17.2 mA
  R_{18}: 34.39 mA
  R_{19}: 6.4 mA
  R_{20}: 21.32 mA
  R_{21}: 21.32 mA
  R_{22}: 7.11 mA
  R_{23}: 7.11 mA
  R_{24}: 7.11 mA
  R_{25}: 21.32 mA

g. $I_1 = 44.28$ mA
  $I_2 = 34.39$ mA
  $I_3 = 21.32$ mA

INSTRUCTIONAL UNIT

Voltage division and current division

This instructional unit is for those who do not yet understand the concepts of voltage division and current division. Comprehension of these two concepts in electronics is very important. The purpose of this unit, therefore, is to present a simplified analogy to electron flow to explain and clarify these concepts.

Voltage, current, and resistance are by now familiar terms. Theoretical physicists have defined them, and students have dutifully memorized the definitions. The purpose of this instructional unit is to make these definitions more meaningful.

Three components essential for voltage division and current division are:

1. Voltage source (for example, transformer or battery)
2. Conductor
3. Resistance

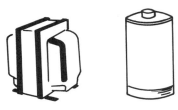

Voltage source

Deviating from the strict definition of physicists and using simple terms, we will discuss the effects resulting from the use of each of the components shown.

A transformer or battery can be used as a voltage source. Voltage is an electrical pressure, that is, a force that pushes electrons through wires.

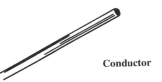

Conductor

The wires permit a current or passage of electrons to flow through the circuit. The wires are conductors of current.

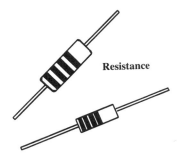

Resistance

Resistance is opposition to the flow of current.

Therefore, there are three components: the battery pushing the electrons, the wire allowing free passage of the electrons, and the resistor making passage of the electrons difficult.

There is one more condition that is required before any of these functions can be accomplished.

Circuit of battery, resistor, and wire

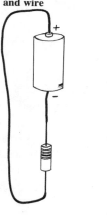

Schematic

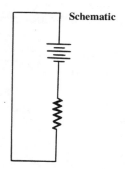

Conceptual presentation

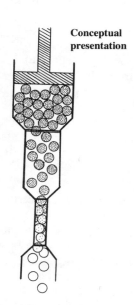

These components must be connected in a closed circuit, that is, the electrons must have a continuous, unbroken pathway from one side of the battery (−) to the other side (+).

In this arrangement of components, the battery voltage pushes the electrons via the conducting wire through the resistor in a steady stream or a constant current.

The schematic representation of the circuit being discussed follows. The symbol for battery is: ⊣⊢. The long vertical line is always the positive pole, and the short vertical line is the negative pole.

The resistor is represented as: —⟋⟍⟋⟍⟋⟍—, and the wires are designated by continuous lines.

The battery forces electrons through the circuit. Once the electrons reach the other side of the battery (+ pole), there is zero force (0 voltage) being exerted upon them. This is what is meant by the expression "voltage drop." The voltage or pushing force on the electrons is used up entirely in the process of pushing the electrons through all resistances in the circuit. This driving force is given up as heat energy as the electrons "squeeze through" the resistor.

A conceptual presentation of what occurs in this simple circuit is shown here. This is a container filled with particles. A plunger is used to push the particles out of the container through a pathway, in which there is a constricted duct, and then on into an open area. The plunger represents the force, and the container is the reservoir of particles. Thus the container and plunger represent the battery. The passageway allowing easy flow of the particles represents the conductor or wire in the schematic. The smaller duct represents a resistance. The open area below the duct represents the positive pole of the battery.

A constant pressure is exerted on the particles. The darkness of the stipple with which the particles are represented is directly proportional to the amount of pressure on each particle (call this "pressure energy"). Notice that as the particles pass *with difficulty* through the duct, each particle loses its "pressure energy." As the particles are pushed through the small

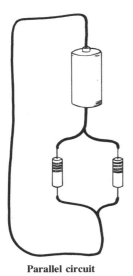

Parallel circuit

duct, the walls of the duct become warm. The particles reaching the open area no longer have any driving force exerted on them.

With this simple circuit and the description of its operation as a basis, we will now discuss the circuit configurations required for current division and for voltage division.

Current division is accomplished in a parallel circuit. A parallel circuit is one in which all positive terminals are connected to a common point and all negative terminals are connected to a second common point.

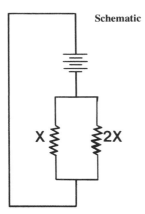

Schematic

Here the previous diagram is represented schematically. The only additional information added to this schematic is that one resistor has 2× the resistance of the other resistor.

In this circuit the voltage drop over each of the resistors is the same. But the current differs. Since one resistor will resist electron flow twice as much as the other, the flow of electrons (current) through the X resistor will be greater than the current through the 2X resistor.

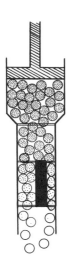

Conceptual presentation

A conceptual view of this circuit includes the container of particles and the passageway leading from the container. The passageway is then divided into two ducts of different sizes. One duct is twice as large as the other. Note that the larger duct allows the passage of twice as many particles as the smaller duct. Thus, the larger duct passes twice as much current as the smaller duct.

The particles arrive at the open area having no stipple or energy. No matter what duct they pass through, they each lose the same amount of energy, that is, there was the same voltage drop through each duct.

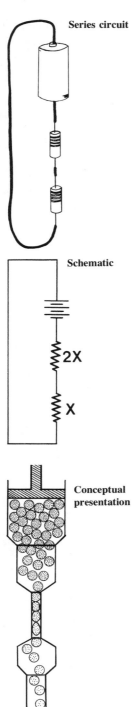

Series circuit

Schematic

2X

X

Conceptual presentation

To achieve a division of voltage, a series configuration is used. In this series circuit, the resistances are connected end-to-end so that the same current flows throughout the circuit.

In this schematic, the resistances are designated X and 2X, that is, 2X has twice the resistance to current flow that X does.

The current is determined by the total resistance in the circuit. The current does not change in this circuit, since there is only one pathway to follow.

However, the voltage is different above the resistors and between the resistors and is zero below the resistors. The total voltage drops over the two resistors, with twice as much lost in the 2X resistor as is lost in the X resistor.

A conceptual view of voltage division is shown. The first duct through which the particles must pass is twice as narrow as the second duct. Therefore, it is twice as difficult for the particles to get by the first duct as it is for them to get by the second. Thus, twice as much voltage or force is required (lost) to get the particles through the first duct as is required to get them through the second.

Note that the current (rate of particle flow) is not greater in one duct or the other. The current is the same throughout the passageway.

We will now briefly review the concepts of voltage division and current division.

Voltage division

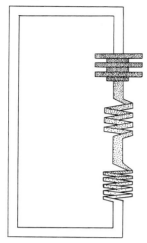

Voltage division occurs when resistances are in a series configuration.

The stipple in the figure indicates voltage; more stipple means higher voltage.

The battery forces electrons through the circuit. The energy of force (voltage) is used up entirely in pushing the electrons through the resistances. The smaller the resistance to electron flow, the smaller the force required to push the electrons through the resistor. The greater the resistance, the greater the voltage required to get the electrons through the resistor. In this figure, the first resistor offers less resistance than the second resistor.

Knowing these facts, turn to p. 56 and answer question 1.

Current division

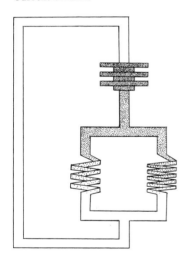

Current division occurs when resistances are in a parallel configuration.

Note that the two resistances are not the same. The one on the left allows easier passage of current than the one on the right. Most electrons will take the route of least resistance; therefore, there will be greater current through the left resistor than through the right resistor.

Note that the force at the top of each of the resistances is the same and that the force at the bottom of each of the resistances is zero. Therefore, the same amount of force was used to push the electrons through each of the resistors.

Refer to p. 56 and answer question 2.

QUESTIONS

1. a. Which resistor will require the greater portion of the force to get the electrons pushed through?
   b. If you required a voltage equal to the battery voltage, what would be a good point from which to obtain that voltage?
   c. If you wanted a voltage less than that of the battery, from what point would you obtain the voltage?
   d. Is the current through the first and the second resistors the same or different?
   e. Are these resistors connected in series or in parallel?
2. a. Are these resistors connected in series or parallel?
   b. Is the current the same through each resistor?
   c. Is the same amount of voltage required to push the electrons through each of the resistors?
   d. What is the voltage below each resistor?

ANSWERS

1. a. Second resistor
   b. Above both resistors
   c. Top of second resistor
   d. Same
   e. Series

2. a. Parallel
   b. No
   c. Yes
   d. Zero

CHAPTER 6

RESISTORS

As shown in previous chapters, strategically placed resistors of specifically selected values can regulate voltages and current flow in a circuit. A resistor is an electronic component that serves the useful function of providing circuits with resistance or hindrance to current flow. Thus, current limitation is achieved through the use of resistors. Resistors come in various types of construction and in many sizes and shapes. Resistors may be classified as fixed or variable. A fixed resistor has only one specified value that is unchanged during normal operation. A variable resistor allows for a selection of resistance within the specified range of the resistor. The most common types of fixed and variable resistors will be discussed.

FIXED RESISTORS

The symbol for a fixed value resistor is ———/\/\/\/\———.

Carbon resistors

The construction of carbon resistors is shown in Fig. 6-1. This resistor is made up of a resistive element, wire leads, an insulative casing, and an outer coating of a moisture-proofing material. The resistive element is composed of a mixture of a conducting material (carbon) and a nonconducting material (resin). The resistance is determined by the proportions of carbon and resin used. With more carbon and less resin, a small amount of resistance is created. A small amount of carbon with a large amount of resin produces a large resistance. It is easy to understand why these carbon resistors are also known as composition

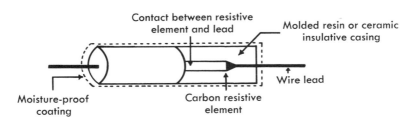

Fig. 6-1. Cutaway view of carbon resistor.

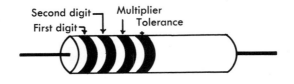

Color	Value	Tolerance	
Black	0	Gold	± 5%
Brown	1	Silver	±10%
Red	2	No band	±20%
Orange	3		
Yellow	4		
Green	5		
Blue	6	Multiplier is the number of zeros added to the first two digits	
Violet	7		
Gray	8		
White	9		

Fig. 6-2. Resistor color code.

resistors, since the resistance depends upon the composition of the resistive element. The composition, not the size, of the resistor determines the value of resistance.

The carbon resistor is constructed in such a way that thickened, fan-shaped ends of the lead wires make good contact with the resistive element and secure the lead wire in place within the insulative casing of the resistor. The casing consists of resin or ceramic. A moisture proof material (for example, wax or lacquer) is used to coat the exterior surface of the resistor.

The physical size of a composition resistor is related not to its resistance value but rather to its wattage rating. The larger the diameter of a resistor, the higher the wattage rating. Increased insulative material and surface area contribute to a resistor's ability to dissipate greater amounts of heat. The relationship between resistor diameter and wattage rating is apparent when you consider that a ⅛ inch resistor has a rating of ½ W, a ¼ inch resistor 1 W, and a 5/16 inch resistor 2 W.

Fixed-value carbon resistors are generally used where power dissipation is low and where precise values of resistance are not needed. The range of values available is approximately 5 Ω to 22 MΩ, with tolerance values of ±5%, ±10%, or ±20%.

An internationally accepted series of colored bands is printed on most resistors to indicate the value of the resistance and the degree of tolerance (Fig. 6-2). Therefore, the value of a resistor can be interpreted from its colorful

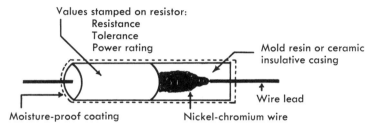

Fig. 6-3. Cutaway view of wire-wound resistor.

striped jacket. The tolerance of a color-coded resistor indicates the maximum percent of deviation from the given value of the resistor that can be expected. The fourth stripe of the color code gives the tolerance, as shown in Fig. 6-2.

Wire-wound resistors

Wire offers a certain amount of resistance to the flow of current. The resistance (ohms) can be calculated if a few dimensions and properties of the wire are known, including radius (r) or cross sectional area ($A = \pi r^2$) in centimeters, length (l) in centimeters, and resistivity (ρ) in ohms. The resistance of a given length of wire of a specific metal composition can be calculated with the equation: $R = \rho l/A$. Thus, if a resistor of a specified value is needed, it can be made by using a calculated length of wire. For space considerations, the length of wire can be compactly arranged by winding the wire tightly around an insulating material.

A wire-wound resistor (Fig. 6-3) consists of nickel-chromium wire tightly wrapped around a central insulating core, leads attached to each end of the nickel-chromium wire, and a casing of insulating and moisture-proofing material (for example, silicone or vitreous enamel). This type of resistor is used where precise values of resistance are needed and/or high power dissipation is required. Wire-wound resistors have excellent stability, can be made with power ratings greater than 200 W, and are available in values up to about 100 kΩ. The values, tolerances, and power ratings are stamped on the resistor.

VARIABLE RESISTORS

Some resistors are designed so that a variable amount of the total resistance can be used. Commonly called *potentiometers,* variable resistors are also known as *rheostats.* In common electronic jargon, a potentiometer is called a "pot," and its symbol is —⋀⋀⋀— . There are two types of potentiometers generally available, nickel-chromium and carbon.

Carbon potentiometer

A carbon potentiometer is constructed by depositing a layer of carbon on a circular strip of insulation (Fig. 6-4). A metal wiper arm that slides on the carbon

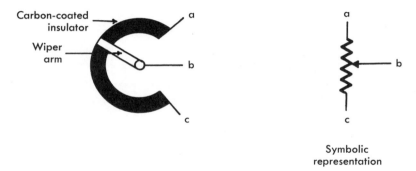

Fig. 6-4. Carbon potentiometer.

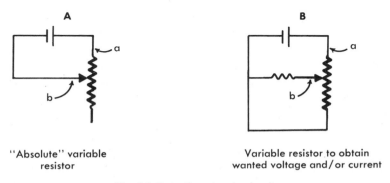

Fig. 6-5. Potentiometers in circuit.

surface provides the point at which the desired resistance is selected. Commonly a specified voltage or a specified current is wanted. The potentiometer can be arranged in a circuit configuration for current selection, voltage selection, or both.

Shown in Fig. 6-5, *A,* is a potentiometer connected so as to absolutely change the battery and point *b* at 0V. Since the voltage drop across the resistor is constant Voltage at points *a* and *b,* however, remains constant, point *a* at the voltage of the battery and point *b* at 0V. Since the voltage drop across the resistor is constant and the resistance is increased, it follows from Ohm's law that the current is decreased. On the other hand, if the wiper arm is moved upward, the resistance will decrease, the voltage drop across the resistor will remain unchanged, and the current will increase.

Fig. 6-5, *B,* represents the more common application of a potentiometer. When the wiper arm is moved, the total resistance of the potentiometer does not change, but the total effective resistance in the circuit does change. For example, if the wiper arm is moved downward, the resistance between points *a* and *b* is increased, which will result in a decrease in voltage at point *b.* The total effective resistance will be increased; therefore, the current in the circuit will be decreased.

Thus, when the wiper arm of the potentiometer is moved, changes in current and voltage result.

Carbon potentiometers are limited to applications requiring low power dissipation and to regulating large resistances. These potentiometers tend to become electrically "noisy" after considerable use. This occurs when the carbon surfaces become rough and the wiper arms become dirty because of loose carbon. In time, some areas of the carbon surface may wear away so that bald patches occur. The carbon surfaces can be cleaned of dirt and loose carbon patches, but the bald spots cannot be repaired. However, replacement carbon potentiometers are relatively inexpensive and easily installed.

Normally the contact between the carbon strip and the wiper arm is not as good as that in a wire-wound potentiometer. Poor contact can result in increased resistance. Therefore, when close regulation of resistance is essential in a circuit, a wire-wound potentiometer is used.

Wire-wound potentiometer

Wire-wound potentiometers are made by closely winding a coil of nickel-chromium wire around a strip of insulating material, all of which is bent into a circular form similar to that of the carbon potentiometer just described. An oxide coating on the wire insulates each turn of the wire, but bare metal is exposed to the wiper arm for good contact.

In addition to this usual shape, the resistive element can be bent into a spiral shape. If the wiper arm is mounted on a screw-threaded shaft, the shaft will gradually move the wiper arm down the spiral. By allowing the entire range of resistance to be covered in many turns (10 or more) of the shaft rather than just one, very small changes in resistance are possible.

Wire-wound potentiometers are made in a vast array of physical sizes and shapes. They are available in values ranging from a few ohms to about 100 kΩ. Power ratings usually vary up to about 3 W. Tolerances range from ±20% to ±1%. The increased stability and accuracy of wire-wound potentiometers make their use desirable.

RESISTORS IN DC AND AC CIRCUITS

Resistance is an opposition to current flow. The resistance exerted by a resistor is independent of the frequency of the electrical signal. Therefore, for all practical purposes, ac and dc are affected in the same way when passed through a resistor.

However, in alternating current circuits, another kind of opposition to current exists, which is called *reactance*. Reactance is caused by the presence of capacitors and inductors (both of which will be discussed later) and is dependent upon the frequency of the electrical signal. The combined current-opposing effect of reactance and resistance in ac circuits is called *impedance*. In other words, electrical hindrance to ac is called impedance. Impedance (Z) in ac circuits is equivalent to resistance (R) in dc circuits. The ohm is the unit of measure of both impedance and resistance.

INSTRUCTIONAL ACTIVITIES

1. a. Display an assortment of different types of resistors, including:
   (1) Carbon resistors of various values and power ratings
   (2) Wire-wound resistors of various values and power ratings
   (3) Carbon potentiometers
   (4) Wire-wound potentiometers
   b. Expose the interior of a representative of each of the four types of resistors to illustrate the construction.
   c. Students are to measure with a VOM the resistance of each of the four types of resistors. This exercise will allow students to establish for themselves how potentiometers must be connected to obtain resistance values.
2. Students are to look at circuits in commonly used instruments and to identify the different types of resistors in those circuits. Students will realize that many adjustable dials on instruments are potentiometers, for example, zero adjust and fine and course adjustments on spectrophotometers.
3. a. Given batteries, carbon resistors, potentiometers, and leads, the students are to build two circuits:
   (1) A circuit in which the potentiometer regulates current but not voltage (refer to Fig. 6-5, *A*)
   (2) A circuit in which the potentiometer regulates both voltage and current (refer to Fig. 6-5, *B*)
   b. Given a VOM, students are to demonstrate the operation of each of the two circuits built.
4. Given a carbon potentiometer and two or three wire-wound potentiometers (for example, one-turn; five-turn; and ten-turn), students are to select the potentiometer most appropriate for:
   a. A fine adjustment in a spectrophotometer
   b. A light dimmer
   c. A course adjustment in a spectrophotometer
   d. A null-balance adjustment (for example, in freezing point depression osmometers or in fluorometers)

PRACTICE PROBLEMS and STUDY QUESTIONS

1. The values and tolerances of carbon resistors are designated by a code of colored bands on the resistor jacket. Given below are colored bands listed in order from the band closest to the end of the resistor. For each resistor give:
   a. Value of the carbon resistor
   b. Percent of tolerance rating
   c. Range of acceptable resistance values
   (1) Red – red – red – silver
   (2) Brown – black – black – gold
   (3) Orange – red – brown – gold
   (4) White – blue – violet – silver
   (5) Gray – black – brown
   (6) Green – green – red – silver
2. For each of the following two circuits, with the wiper arm at each of the first five numbered positions (each position equals 2 kΩ), calculate:
   a. Total effective resistance
   b. Voltage at points *a* and *b*
   c. Current flowing past points *a* and *b*

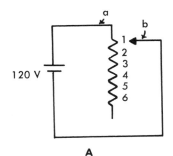

A

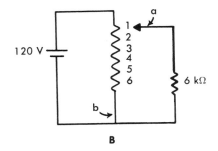

B

ANSWERS

1. (1) a. 2200 Ω or 2.2 kΩ   b. 10%   c. 1980 Ω to 2420 Ω
  (2) a. 10 Ω   b. 5%   c. 9.5 Ω to 10.5 Ω
  (3) a. 320 Ω   b. 5%   c. 304 Ω to 336 Ω
  (4) a. 960 MΩ   b. 10%   c. 864 MΩ to 1056 MΩ
  (5) a. 800 Ω   b. 20%   c. 640 Ω to 960 Ω
  (6) a. 5.5 kΩ   b. 10%   c. 4.95 kΩ to 6.05 kΩ

2. A 1. a. 2 kΩ   b. a = 120 V   b = 0 V   c. 60 mA at a and b
    2. a. 4 kΩ   b. a = 120 V   b = 0 V   c. 30 mA at a and b
    3. a. 6 kΩ   b. a = 120 V   b = 0 V   c. 20 mA at a and b
    4. a. 8 kΩ   b. a = 120 V   b = 0 V   c. 15 mA at a and b
    5. a. 10 kΩ   b. a = 120 V   b = 0 V   c. 12 mA at a and b
  B 1. a. 5.75 kΩ   b. a = 78.26 V   b = 0 V   c. a = 13.04 mA   b = 7.23 mA
    2. a. 7.43 kΩ   b. a = 55.4 V   b = 0 V   c. a = 9.23 mA   b = 6.92 mA
    3. a. 9.0 kΩ   b. a = 40.0 V   b = 0 V   c. a = 6.67 mA   b = 6.67 mA
    4. a. 10.4 kΩ   b. a = 27.7 V   b = 0 V   c. a = 4.62 mA   b = 6.92 mA
    5. a. 11.5 kΩ   b. a = 15.65 V   b = 0 V   c. a = 2.60 mA   b = 7.82 mA

APPROACH TO SOLVING PROBLEMS

2. A 1. a. 2 kΩ
    2. a. 2 kΩ + 2 kΩ = 4 kΩ
    3. a. 2 kΩ + 2 kΩ + 2 kΩ = 6 kV
    4. a. 2 kΩ + 2 kΩ + 2 kΩ + 2 kΩ = 8 kΩ
    5. a. 2 kΩ + 2 kΩ + 2 kΩ + 2 kΩ + 2 kΩ = 10 kΩ

    1. b. to 5. b. Point b is negative side of battery; therefore = 0 V.

    1. c. I = E/R = 120 V/2 kΩ = 60 mA at a and b
    2. c. I = E/R = 120 V/4 kΩ = 30 mA at a and b
    3. c. I = E/R = 120 V/6 kΩ = 20 mA at a and b
    4. c. I = E/R = 120 V/8 kΩ = 15 mA at a and b
    5. c. I = E/R = 120 V/10 kΩ = 12 mA at a and b

  B 1. a. 2 kΩ + 3.75 kΩ = 5.75 kΩ
    2. a. 4 kΩ + 3.43 kΩ = 7.43 kΩ
    3. a. 6 kΩ + 3 kΩ = 9 kΩ
    4. a. 8 kΩ + 2.4 kΩ = 10.4 kΩ
    5. a. 10 kΩ + 1.5 kΩ = 11.5 kΩ

    1. b. a:(120 V) − [(2 kΩ/5.75 kΩ) (120 V)] = 120 V − 41.74 V = 78.26 V
    2. b. a:(120 V) − [(4 kΩ/7.43 kΩ) (120 V)] = 120 V − 64.60 V = 55.4 V
    3. b. a:(120 V) − [(6 kΩ/9 kΩ) (120 V)] = 120 V − 80 V = 40 V
    4. b. a:(120 V) − [(8 kΩ/10.4 kΩ) (120 V)] = 120 V − 93.2 V = 27.7 V
    5. b. a:(120 V) − [(10 kΩ/11.5 kΩ) (120 V)] = 120 V − 104.35 V = 15.65 V

    1. c. a:I = E/R = 78.26 V/6 kΩ = 13.04 mA
       b:I = E/R = 72.26 V/10 kΩ = 7.23 mA
    2. c. a:I = E/R = 55.4 V/6 kΩ = 9.23 mA
       b:I = E/R = 55.4 V/8 kΩ = 6.92 mA
    3. c. a:I = E/R = 40 V/6 kΩ = 6.67 mA

$$\text{b:} I = E/R = 40 \text{ V}/6 \text{ k}\Omega = 6.67 \text{ mA}$$
$$4. \text{ c. a:} I = E/R = 27.7 \text{ V}/6 \text{ k}\Omega = 4.62 \text{ mA}$$
$$\text{b:} I = E/R = 27.7 \text{ V}/4 \text{ k}\Omega = 6.92 \text{ mA}$$
$$5. \text{ c. a:} I = E/R = 15.65 \text{ V}/6 \text{ k}\Omega = 2.60 \text{ mA}$$
$$\text{b:} I = E/R = 15.65 \text{ V}/2 \text{ k}\Omega = 7.82 \text{ mA}$$

CHAPTER 7

CAPACITORS

A capacitor is a device used to store a quantity of electrical charge. In its simplest form, it consists of two thin sheets of conducting material separated by a layer of insulating, or dielectric, material. The simplicity of design, as with most common electronic components, is remarkable in light of the considerable importance of its function to particular circuits. Construction is only one of the many factors to be considered in the examination of capacitors. Functions and characteristics of capacitors to be presented in this section include: storage of a charge, units of and factors affecting capacitance, common types and voltage ratings of capacitors, capacitors in series and parallel, charging and discharging time constants, phase relationship, and capacitive reactance.

HOW A CAPACITOR STORES A CHARGE

A representation of a capacitor with no potential placed across it is shown in Fig. 7-1, *A*. The switch (S) is open; therefore, current does not flow. The layer of insulation between the plates is called a *dielectric,* for which commonly used materials include air, plastic, mica, ceramic, and wax-saturated paper. As noted in Chapter 2, insulators consist of atoms in which the electrons are tightly held in their orbits.

When the switch is closed (Fig. 7-1, *B*), current flows instantly but for only a brief time. Conventional current flows from a higher positive potential to a lower positive potential. Therefore, in the wire connecting the positive terminal of the battery to the capacitor, the current flows from the battery to the capacitor plate, and in the wire connecting the capacitor to the negative terminal, the current flows from the capacitor to the negative terminal. The dielectric does not conduct a current, that is, the current does not pass through the capacitor. As a result, current flows only as long as there is a potential difference between the capacitor plates and the battery terminals to which they are connected. Once the potential on the plates equals the potential of the battery, current no longer flows and the capacitor is said to be charged.

The charge on the plates exerts a force on the atoms in the dielectric. The electrons in the dielectric atoms are attracted by the positively charged plate and repelled by the negatively charged plate, resulting in the orbital distortion shown

65

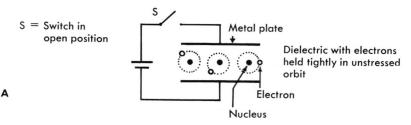

S = Switch in
     open position

A

Capacitor with no charge on its plates

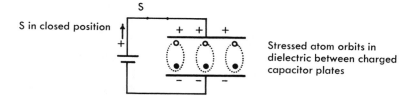

S in closed position

B

Charging of a capacitor

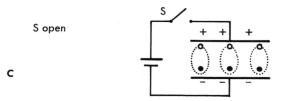

S open

C

Charged capacitor in open circuit

Fig. 7-1. Storage of a charge on a capacitor.

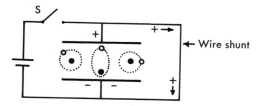

Fig. 7-2. Discharging capacitor.

in Fig. 7-1, *B*. The force exerted between the charged plates and the atoms in the dielectric is called an *electrostatic field* and is effective in holding the charge on the capacitor plates even after the switch is opened (Fig. 7-1, *C*). This charged capacitor is essentially a dc voltage source ready to be discharged.

The capacitor can be discharged by providing a completed pathway or shunt from the positive to the negative side of the capacitor (Fig. 7-2). The potential difference across the capacitor causes a current to flow through the wire shunt from the positive to the negative side of the capacitor. Current flows until there is no longer a potential across the capacitor. Once completely discharged, the dielectric atoms will have their original unstressed circular orbits. The charging rate of a capacitor can be regulated by selecting a resistor through which to pass the charging current. Likewise, the discharging rate can be regulated by inserting a resistor in place of the wire shunt shown in Fig. 7-2. Charging and discharging rates will be discussed in greater detail later in this chapter.

In summary, when a dc voltage is placed across a capacitor, current flows briefly even though there is not a completed circuit. (There is no complete circuit for dc because there is a break in the continuity of the conducting material caused by an insulator.) Current flows until the two plates attain the potential of the battery, that is, until the capacitor is charged. When the capacitor is charged, electrical energy is stored in an electrostatic field set up in the dielectric by distorting electron orbits. When the capacitor is discharging, the energy stored in the dielectric is released in the form of current flow.

UNITS OF CAPACITANCE

The ability of a capacitor to store an electrical charge is called capacitance. The abbreviation for capacitance is C. The symbols used to represent capacitors in schematics are shown below. When the symbols on the right are used, the curved side represents the plate connected either to ground or to the low voltage side of the circuit.

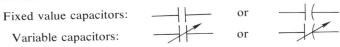

The unit of capacitance is the *farad*, abbreviated F. One farad is the capacitance that stores one coulomb of electrical energy when one volt is applied. Recall that a coulomb is a unit of measure of the quantity of an electric charge that is equal to the combined charges of 6.28×10^{18} electrons. In more practical terms, a coulomb is equal to one ampere of current flowing past a point in one second. The equation used to calculate capacitance is:

$$C \text{ (farads)} = Q \text{ (coulombs)}/V \text{ (volts)}$$

The farad is too large for most applications. Units commonly used are either the microfarad, designated μF (a millionth of a farad or 10^{-6} farad), or the picofarad, designated pF (a millionth of a microfarad or 10^{-12} farad).

FACTORS AFFECTING CAPACITANCE

The capacitance of a capacitor is determined by the area of and the distance between the plates and by the dielectric material used. The ability of a capacitor to store electrical energy depends upon the electrostatic field established between the plates and the degree of distortion of the electron orbits of the dielectric atoms. Increasing the area of the plates exposes more dielectric to the distortion effects of the electrostatic field and therefore increases the capacitance. Furthermore, if the dielectric layer is made very thin, bringing the plates closer together, the electrostatic field will be intensified, thus increasing the capacitance. Finally,

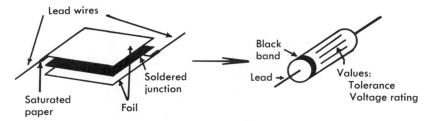

Fig. 7-3. Construction of a paper capacitor.

the material used as a dielectric influences the amount of capacitance obtained. The degree of distortion of the electron orbits of the dielectric varies with the material used. Air is used as the reference material and is said to have a dielectric constant of 1. Other substances may have higher dielectric constants, meaning that their atoms undergo greater distortion under similar circumstances. Increased distortion yields higher capacitance for the same thickness of material. For example, under similar conditions, a layer of mica will have a dielectric constant of 6 compared to the same thickness of air. Thus a capacitor using mica as the dielectric has a capacitance six times as great as an identical capacitor using air as the dielectric. Paper has a dielectric constant of 2 or 3. Titanium oxide has a very high dielectric constant of over 150 times that of an equivalent layer of air.

COMMON TYPES OF CAPACITORS
Fixed capacitors

1. The tubular paper capacitor is the most common type. It consists of a strip of paper saturated with any one of a variety of materials, such as petroleum jelly or paraffin wax, sandwiched between strips of metal foil. Commonly the metal foil used is aluminum.

Fig. 7-3 shows a common way of making a paper capacitor. A sheet of impregnated paper is placed between two sheets of aluminum foil. Protruding from the foil are tabs that are soldered to the lead wires for contact to the external circuit. The three sheets are rolled up to conserve space, and the entire unit is sealed to protect against moisture, to insulate, and to give mechanical stability. A black band is usually painted on the end at which the lead is connected to the outside layer of foil. Values, tolerance, and voltage rating are stamped on the surface. This type of capacitor is available in sizes from a few pF to 100 μF. Tolerances generally range from ±10% to ±25%.

2. A mica capacitor is a fixed-value capacitor that uses mica as the dielectric between plates of metal, usually silver. These capacitors are very efficient and reliable but are expensive. Fig. 7-4 shows their general construction. Because mica is brittle and like a multilayered sandwich, it cannot be rolled. Alternate silver plates are connected together and attached to a lead wire. The capacitor is usually encased in molded Bakelite. Mica capacitors are usually available in values from a few pF to about 10,000 pF and can be made to a tolerance of ±2%.

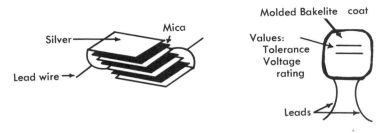

Fig. 7-4. Construction of a mica capacitor.

The two types of capacitors described above are representative of fixed-value, "dry" capacitors. When larger capacitances are needed, another type of capacitor is usually employed, the so-called "wet" or electrolytic capacitor.

3. One example of the wet type of capacitor consists of a loosely rolled or folded sheet of aluminum that is immersed in a borax solution (electrolyte). The borax solution causes an extremely thin layer of aluminum oxide and oxygen gas to form on the surface of the aluminum. The aluminum sheet becomes one plate of the capacitor, and the borax solution becomes the other plate. The layer of aluminum oxide and oxygen will not conduct electricity and therefore becomes the dielectric. Because this dielectric layer is extremely thin, the capacitance is increased greatly. The aluminum plate side of the capacitor must always be connected to the positive side of the circuit. If the aluminum plate side of the capacitor is connected to the negative side of the circuit, the dielectric will be "punctured" by the current when the metal plate becomes negative, and the capacitance will be destroyed. Although "wet" type capacitors are self-healing (in other words, if the proper connections are made, a new coating of oxide and gas will form), once a capacitor has been misused, it should be discarded.

4. A variation of the above capacitor, which avoids having to handle a device containing a volume of liquid that may spill, is to replace the solution with a wet cloth. A cloth strip is saturated with borax solution, placed on the metal strip, and rolled up. Electrolytic capacitors are more expensive than the dry capacitors. Electrolytic capacitors are available in a value range of 1 to 5,000 μF and generally have tolerances of -20% to $+50\%$.

5. Another type of electrolytic capacitor substitutes tantalum foil for aluminum, providing more stability, less "noise," and less "leakage current." Although made up like the aluminum type, tantalum foil capacitors rarely employ liquids, can be completely sealed, and are generally physically smaller than aluminum electrolytic capacitors of similar value.

Variable capacitors

Some circuit functions require capacitors with adjustable values of capacitance. There are two general types of variable capacitors. In one, the effective area of the plates can be adjusted; in the other, the distance between plates can be adjusted. Both types use metal (usually aluminum) plates and air as the dielectric.

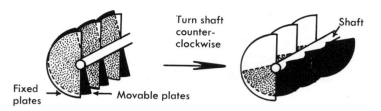

Fig. 7-5. Variable capacitor.

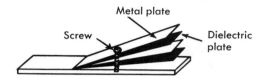

Fig. 7-6. Variable capacitor.

1. Adjustment of plate area can be accomplished by an arrangement of stationary and movable semicircular plates positioned alternately. The movable plates are attached to a rotating shaft. As the shaft is turned, the area of the plates facing each other is changed (Fig. 7-5). Additional variable area can be obtained by increasing the number of plates used in the construction of this type of capacitor. Since the area of the plates can be adjusted, the capacitance of the capacitor can be varied. (This type of capacitor is frequently used as the control to select stations on a radio.)

2. The other type of variable capacitor is one that changes the distance between plates. Fig. 7-6 shows the general construction. A number of metal plates are sandwiched between layers of dielectric material (air). The metal plates are constructed so they will spread apart. An insulated screw through all the plates can compress or allow the plates to flare open. Changing the distance between the plates changes the capacitance.

VOLTAGE RATING OF CAPACITORS

There are restrictions on the conditions under which capacitors can be used. Some of the features of the dielectric material influence the degree of capacitance. The dielectric also serves as a thin layer of insulation between the capacitor plates. All capacitors are given a voltage rating that is the maximum dc voltage that can be used safely without exceeding the insulating capability of the dielectric. When a certain level of voltage is exceeded, an arc of current will flow, causing a "breakdown" or "puncture" of the capacitor. The "working voltage" of a capacitor depends upon the dielectric material used. It must be remembered that when a capacitor is used in an ac line, ac voltages are usually given in rms values. If, for example, a capacitor is rated at 400 working volts dc, 400 volts ac cannot be placed across it.

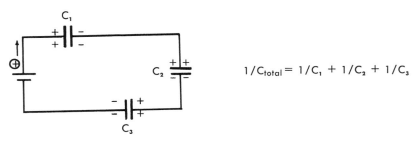

Fig. 7-7. Three capacitors in series.

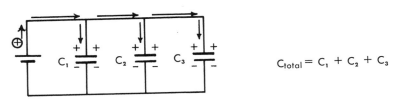

Fig. 7-8. Three capacitors in parallel.

CAPACITORS IN SERIES AND PARALLEL

The rules for adding capacitances in series and parallel circuits are the opposite of those for adding resistances.

Series: For any number of capacitors connected in series, the total or equivalent capacitance is:

$$1/C_{total} = 1/C_1 + 1/C_2 + 1/C_3 \ldots 1/C_n$$

Fig. 7-7 shows three capacitors connected in series across a battery. The positive charge from the positive side of the battery flows to C_1, placing a positive charge on the plate nearest the positive terminal of the battery. The positive charge on the left plate of C_3 moves to the negative side of the battery, leaving a negative charge on the left plate of C_2 and, therefore, a positive charge on the right plate of C_3 and a negative charge on the lower plate of C_2. The electrons move from the upper plate of C_2 to the right plate of C_1, leaving the upper plate of C_2 positive and the right plate of C_1 negative.

Parallel: For any number of capacitors connected in parallel, the total capacitance is simply the sum of all the individual capacitances:

$$C_{total} = C_1 + C_2 + C_3 \ldots C_n$$

Fig. 7-8 shows a parallel arrangement of capacitors.

RESISTANCE-CAPACITANCE TIME CONSTANTS
Charging time constant

If a capacitor is placed directly across a source of voltage with no resistance in the circuit, the capacitor is charged to its full extent in an extremely short period of time. However, a resistor placed in series with a capacitor limits the

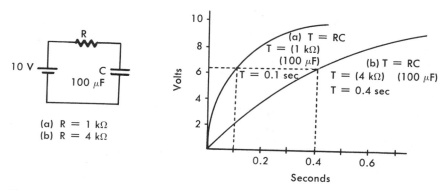

Fig. 7-9. RC charging time constant; affected by value of resistor in series with capacitor.

current flow and, therefore, the charging of the capacitor takes a longer period of time. (Theoretically, with resistance in the circuit, the capacitor never quite reaches full charge.)

The time constant of a capacitor is, by definition, the time in seconds required for a capacitor to reach 63% of full charge, that is, 63% of the applied voltage. The time necessary to reach this 63% level depends upon the amounts of resistance and capacitance. The equation for determining the time constant is:

$T = RC$

where:

   T = Time constant in seconds
   C = Capacitance in farads
   R = Resistance in ohms

Thus, if C is expressed in farads and R in ohms, the time constant is in seconds. If C is expressed in microfarads and R in megohms, the time constant is again expressed in seconds.

Example:

   $R = 4\ M\Omega$
   $C = 0.02\ \mu F$
   $T = RC = (4\ M\Omega)\ (0.02\ \mu F) = 0.8\ sec$

Thus, in 0.08 sec, a 0.02-μF capacitor will charge up to 63% of the supply voltage that is connected across it and the 4 MΩ resistor. Refer to Fig. 7-9.

Discharging time constant

If the charged capacitor is connected in a closed conducting circuit, the potential on the capacitor will cause a current to flow from the positive to the negative plates of the capacitor. Thus, a resistor connected in parallel with the capacitor will determine the time required for the capacitor to discharge. This RC discharge time is calculated with the same equation used to calculate the RC charging time constant. Refer to Fig. 7-10.

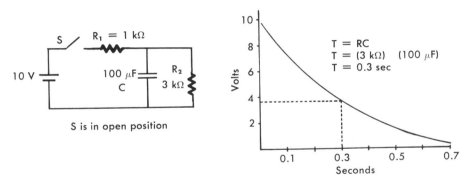

Fig. 7-10. Discharge of a capacitor.

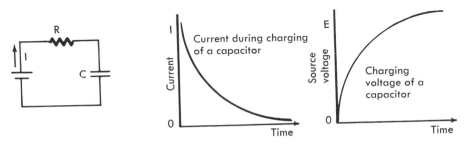

Fig. 7-11. Voltage and current in dc circuit during charging of a capacitor.

PHASE RELATIONSHIP

With the initial application of a dc potential across an uncharged capacitor, there is a maximum current flow and a minimum potential stored on the capacitor. As a charge collects on the plates of the capacitor, the current decreases. In other words, as voltage on the capacitor increases, it exerts a reversed force (back EMF) that decreases current flow. When the capacitor is fully charged, the back EMF equals the EMF of the battery, and no current flows. This phenomenon is shown in Fig. 7-11.

When an ac voltage is applied across a capacitor, the capacitor alternately charges and discharges. The capacitor is charged by the peak voltage of the ac signal (Fig. 7-12, *A* and *D*). When the ac signal's amplitude decreases (Fig. 7-12, *B*) and changes polarity (Fig. 7-12, *C*), the capacitor releases its charge in a direction opposite to the direction of the charging current. The phase relationship of voltage and current in an ac capacitive circuit is that current always leads voltage by 90 degrees. That is, current flows to the capacitor first, and then voltage collects on the capacitor (Fig. 7-13).

CAPACITIVE REACTANCE

Capacitive reactance (X_C) is the resistance to current exerted by a capacitor. As stated earlier, resistance to alternating current is called impedance (Z). Thus,

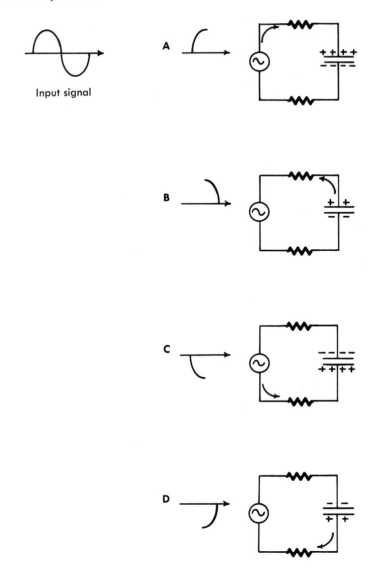

Input signal

Fig. 7-12. Capacitor in ac circuit; effect each quarter sine wave has on a capacitor.

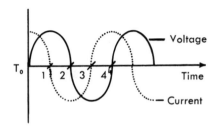

Fig. 7-13. Graphic presentation of voltage and current in capacitive circuit with ac voltage applied.

capacitive reactance and impedance are interchangeable terms, and the ohm remains the unit of measurement.

A capacitor exerts infinite resistance in a dc circuit once the capacitor is charged. The charged capacitor exhibits an infinite reactance, since the back EMF of the capacitor equals the EMF of the voltage source.

In an ac circuit, just as the capacitor begins to become fully charged, the source voltage begins to drop, and the capacitor begins to discharge. If the speed at which the current changes direction is increased (increased frequency), the capacitor has less time to reach a full charge and in fact will not be able to do so. If it cannot reach full charge, it cannot establish a counter EMF equal to the source. In effect, there is less hindrance to current flow as the frequency increases. The relationship of capacitive reactance to frequency is:

$$X_C = 1/2\pi fC$$

where:

X_C = Capacitive reactance in ohms
π = A constant of 3.14
f = Frequency of current in cycles per second
C = Capacitance in farads

To fully appreciate the meaning of this equation, observe the effect on capacitive reactance when the frequency of the ac is changed.

What would the capacitive reactance of a 200 μF capacitor be if applied across it is a 120 Vac signal having a frequency of:
  1. 50 Hz
  2. 100 Hz
  3. 200 Hz

Solutions:

$$X_C = 1/2\pi fC$$
1. $X_C = 1/(2)(3.14)(50 \text{ Hz})(0.0002) = 15.92\ \Omega$
2. $X_C = 1/(2)(3.14)(100 \text{ Hz})(0.0002) = 7.96\ \Omega$
3. $X_C = 1/(2)(3.14)(200 \text{ Hz})(0.0002) = 3.98\ \Omega$

In a purely capacitive circuit, capacitive reactance (X_C) can be substituted for the term impedance in $Z = E/I$, so that Ohm's law for ac circuits becomes:

$$X_C = E/I$$

In a circuit that contains both capacitors and resistors in series, the total impedance is:

$$Z = \sqrt{R^2 + X_C^2}$$

Resistance and capacitive reactance in parallel are added by using the equation:

$$Z = 1/\sqrt{(1/R)^2 + (1/X_C)^2}$$

INSTRUCTIONAL ACTIVITIES

1. Display different types of capacitors (for example, tubular paper, mica, and electrolytic). If old discarded capacitors are available, expose the construction of each type.
2. Students are to identify the different types of capacitors in the circuits of commonly used instruments.
3. Build the RC circuit shown below. For each of the different resistors switched into the circuit:
   a. Use an oscilloscope to monitor charging or discharging of the capacitor
   b. Use the ammeter to monitor current flow
   c. Use a stopwatch to measure RC charging and discharging time (63% of full charge)
   d. Calculate RC times and compare them to the measured RC times

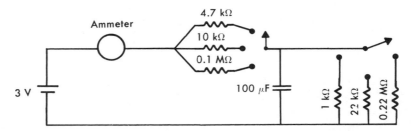

RC charging time constants:

$$4.7 \text{ k}\Omega \times 100 \text{ } \mu\text{F} = 0.47 \text{ sec}$$
$$10 \text{ k}\Omega \times 100 \text{ } \mu\text{F} = 1.0 \text{ sec}$$
$$0.1 \text{ M}\Omega \times 100 \text{ } \mu\text{F} = 10.0 \text{ sec}$$

RC discharging time constants:

$$1 \text{ k}\Omega \times 100 \text{ } \mu\text{F} = 0.1 \text{ sec}$$
$$22 \text{ k}\Omega \times 100 \text{ } \mu\text{F} = 2.2 \text{ sec}$$
$$0.22 \text{ M}\Omega \times 100 \text{ } \mu\text{F} = 22 \text{ sec}$$

PRACTICE PROBLEMS and STUDY QUESTIONS

1. A 3 MΩ resistor and a 5 μF capacitor are connected in series with a 100 V dc source.
   a. What is the time constant for charging the capacitor?
   b. At the end of the charging time calculated in a., what voltage is stored on the capacitor?
2. What is the capacitive reactance of a 150 μF capacitor in a circuit to which is applied 120 Vac at 60 Hz?
3. What is the capacitive reactance of a 100 μF capacitor when a 120 Hz ac voltage is applied?
4. Calculate the total impedance of the following circuits.

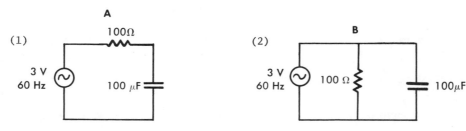

5. Given: Capacitance of a capacitor = 159 μF
           Frequency of ac passing through the capacitor = 1000 Hz
   a. What is the capacitive reactance of the capacitor?
   b. What is the impedance offered by the capacitor?
6. If the voltage rating on a capacitor is 200 Vac ac, what rms value of ac voltage can safely be applied to this capacitor?

7.

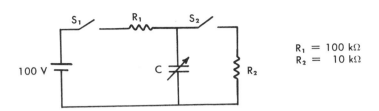

$R_1 = 100 \text{ k}\Omega$
$R_2 = 10 \text{ k}\Omega$

a. If S_1 is closed and S_2 is open, at what value of capacitance must the capacitor (C) be set to obtain a charging time constant of 1 sec?
b. At the end of 1 sec, what voltage is stored on the capacitor (C)?
c. When S_1 is open and S_2 is closed, what is the discharge time constant in this circuit if C is set at 50 μF?

8.

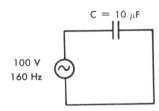

$C = 10 \ \mu F$

100 V
160 Hz

a. What is the current in the circuit above?
b. If the power source were replaced with a 10 Volt battery, what current would flow in the circuit?
9. Given: Capacitors $C_1 = 4 \ \mu F$ and $C_2 = 6 \ \mu F$
   a. What is the total capacitance when C_1 and C_2 are connected in parallel?
   b. What is the total capacitance when C_1 and C_2 are connected in series?
10. Calculate the total impedance in an ac circuit including a 5 μF capacitor in series with a 150 Ω resistor when the frequency of the applied 120 V is:
    a. 100 Hz
    b. 500 Hz
    c. 1000 Hz
11. Calculate the total impedance in an ac circuit in which a 100 μF capacitor is connected in parallel with a 500 Ω resistor when the frequency of the applied 62 V is:
    a. 40 Hz
    b. 200 Hz
    c. 600 Hz

ANSWERS

1. a. 15 sec
   b. 63 V
2. 17.7 Ω
3. 13.3 Ω
4. a. 103.46 Ω
   b. 0.039 Ω
5. a. 1 Ω
   b. 1 Ω
6. 141.4 V
7. a. 10 μF
   b. 63 V
   c. 0.5 sec

8. a. 1.005 A
   b. 0 A
9. a. 10 μF
   b. 2.4 μF
10. a. 150 Ω
    b. 150 Ω
    c. 150 Ω
11. a. 1,574.8 Ω
    b. 7.02 Ω
    c. 63.35 Ω

APPROACH TO SOLVING PROBLEMS

1. a. $T = RC = (3\ M\Omega)(5\ \mu F) = 15\ sec$
   b. 63% of 100 V = 63 V
2. $X_C = 1/2\pi fC = 1/(6.28)(60)(0.00015) = 17.7\ \Omega$
3. $X_C = 1/2\pi fC = 1/(6.28)(120)(0.0001) = 13.3\ \Omega$
4. a. $X_C = 1/2\pi fC = 1/(6.28)(60)(100 \times 10^{-6}) = 26.54\ \Omega$

   $Z = \sqrt{R^2 + X_C^2} = \sqrt{100^2 + (26.54)^2} = \sqrt{10704} = 103.46\ \Omega$

   b. $Z = \sqrt{(1/R)^2 + (1/X_C)^2} = \sqrt{(1/100)^2 + (1/26.54)^2}$

   $= \sqrt{0.001 + 0.0014} = \sqrt{0.0015} = 0.039\ \Omega$

5. a. $X_C = 1/2\pi fC = 1/(6.28)(1000)(0.000159) = 1\ \Omega$
   b. Same as a.
6. rms = (peak voltage)(0.707) = (200 V)(0.707) = 141.4 V
7. a. $C = T/R = 1\ sec/100\ k\Omega = 10\ \mu F$
   b. 63% of 100 = 63 V
   c. $T = RC = (10\ k\Omega)(50\ \mu F) = 0.5\ sec$
8. a. $X_C = 1/2\pi fC = 1/(6.28)(160)(0.00001) = 99.52\ \Omega$
      $I = E/R = 100\ V/99.52\ \Omega = 1.005\ A$
   b. 0 A (a capacitor gives infinite resistance to dc)
9. a. $C_{total} = C_1 + C_2 = 4\ \mu F + 6\ \mu F = 10\ \mu F$
   b. $C_{total} = (C_1)(C_2)/(C_1) + (C_2) = (6\ \mu F)(4\ \mu F)/(6\ \mu F) + (4\ \mu F) = 24\ \mu F/10\ \mu F = 2.4\ \mu F$
10. a. $X_C = 1/2\pi fC = 1/(2)(3.14)(100\ Hz)(0.005\ F) = 1/3.14 = 0.32\ \Omega$

    $Z = \sqrt{R^2 + X_C^2} = \sqrt{150^2 + 0.32^2} = \sqrt{22500 + 0.10}$

    $= \sqrt{22500.1} = 150\ \Omega$

    b. $X_C = 1/2\pi fC = 1/(2)(3.14)(500\ Hz)(0.005\ F) = 1/15.7 = 0.06\ \Omega$

    $Z = \sqrt{R^2 + X_C^2} = \sqrt{150^2 + 0.06^2} = \sqrt{22500 + 0.0036}$

    $= \sqrt{22500} = 150\ \Omega$

    c. $X_C = 1/2\pi fC = 1/(2)(3.14)(1000\ Hz)(0.005\ F) = 1/31.4 = 0.03\ \Omega$

    $Z = \sqrt{R^2 + X_C^2} = \sqrt{150^2 + 0.03^2} = \sqrt{22500 + 0.0009}$

    $= \sqrt{22500} = 150\ \Omega$

11. a. $X_C = 1/2\pi fC = 1/(2)(3.14)(40\ Hz)(0.0001\ F) = 1/0.02512 = 39.81\ \Omega$

    $Z = 1/\sqrt{(1/R)^2 + (1/X_C)^2} = 1/\sqrt{(1/500)^2 + (1/39.81)^2}$

    $= 1/0.000004 + 0.000631 = 1/0.000635 = 1574.8\ \Omega$

    b. $X_C = 1/2\pi fC = 1/(2)(3.14)(200\ Hz)(0.0001\ F) = 1/0.1256 = 7.96\ \Omega$

    $Z = 1/\sqrt{(1/R)^2 + (1/X_C)^2} = 1/\sqrt{(1/500)^2 + (1/7.96)^2}$

    $= 1/0.000004 + 0.015782 = 1/0.015786 = 63.35\ \Omega$

    c. $X_C = 1/2\pi fC = 1/(2)(3.14)(600\ Hz)(0.001\ F) = 1/0.3768 = 2.65\ \Omega$

    $Z = 1/\sqrt{(1/R)^2 + (1/X_C)^2} = 1/\sqrt{(1/500)^2 + (1/2.65)^2}$

    $= 1/0.000004 + 0.142399 = 1/0.142403 = 7.02\ \Omega$

CHAPTER 8

INDUCTORS

A straight wire will conduct a current in a closed circuit. The current is hindered by the resistance offered by the metal wire. However, when the same straight metal wire is coiled, the resistance of the wire is not the only opposition to current flow. What mysterious change results from the new arrangement of the wire? Do charges naturally decelerate in a turn in the conducting "roadway"? Do both dc and ac meet more resistance or impedance in a coiled wire than in a straight wire? What purpose is served by coiling a wire?

ELECTRICITY AND MAGNETISM

Before attempting to answer any of the above questions, consider a straight conducting metal wire in which there exists an invisible force of electricity. This invisible force of electricity has an invisible partner called *magnetism*. When a current is flowing through a conductor, a *magnetic field* surrounds the conductor. The strength of this magnetic field is directly proportional to the quantity of current passing through the conductor and inversely proportional to the distance of the field from the conductor. Magnetic lines of force exist around a *conducting* wire, but when the wire stops conducting the magnetic field collapses.

The lines of force around the current-carrying conductor travel in a clockwise or counter-clockwise direction, depending upon the direction of current flow. The *right hand rule* expresses the direction of magnetic lines of force in relation to the direction of current flow (when referring to conventional current).

Right hand rule: If you grasp a conductor with your right hand with the thumb pointing in the direction of current flow, your fingers will indicate the direction of the magnetic lines of force.

(*Note:* This is called the *left hand rule* if current flow is defined as electron flow. If you grasp a conductor with your left hand with the thumb pointing in the direction of electron flow, your fingers will indicate the direction of the magnetic lines of force.)

Application of the right hand rule to Fig. 8-1 illustrates that a change in the direction of current flow reverses the direction of the magnetic lines of force around the conductor.

79

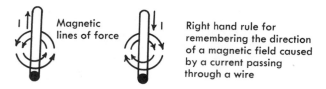

Magnetic lines of force

Right hand rule for remembering the direction of a magnetic field caused by a current passing through a wire

Fig. 8-1. Right hand rule.

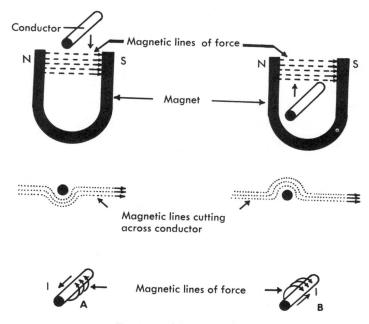

Conductor

Magnetic lines of force

Magnet

Magnetic lines cutting across conductor

Magnetic lines of force

Fig. 8-2. Induction of current.

INDUCTION OF CURRENT

If a current can and does cause a magnetic field, can a magnetic field cause a current? Yes. When magnetic lines of force cut across a conductor, a current is caused to flow or, in other words, a current is induced. Induction of current can be demonstrated with a magnetic field and a conductor. Fig. 8-2 shows the induction of current. The wire can be kept stationary and the magnet moved so that the magnetic lines of force cut across the conductor to induce the current. Or the magnet can be kept stationary and the conductor moved so as to cross perpendicularly the lines of magnetic force, cutting them in a downward (*A*) or an upward (*B*) motion.

Any conductor carrying a current develops magnetic lines of force around it. This magnetic field becomes stronger with increased current and weaker with decreased current and completely collapses when current ceases to flow. This "envelope of magnetic force" can be considered a package of reserved energy, which can be converted to current flow, as shown in Fig. 8-2, if the lines of force

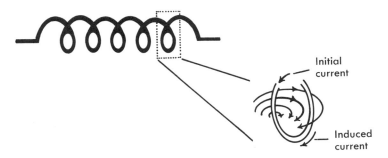

Fig. 8-3. Induced counter EMF.

cut across a conductor. Although these magnetic lines of force exist around a current-conducting straight wire, their presence does not have any appreciable effect on current flow and therefore is ignored. However, magnetic lines of force can have desirable effects on current flow in a circuit if the current passes through a coiled conductor called an inductor or coil.

The symbol for an inductor is ⎓⎓⎓⎓⎓. This inductor does not have a central core other than air; therefore, it is called an air-core inductor. The symbol for an inductor with a central core of iron is ⎓⎓⎓⎓⎓. Variable inductors are shown by one of the following two symbols:

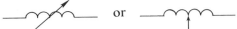

Capacitors and inductors are referred to as *reactors* because they do not dissipate electrical energy in the form of heat, as resistors do, but alternately store energy and then deliver it back to the circuit. Capacitors store energy in an electrostatic field. Inductors store energy in an electromagnetic field. Time is required to accumulate, store, and then release energy. This explains why reactors produce changes in phase relationships between current and voltage.

INDUCTOR IN A DC CIRCUIT

First consideration will be given to direct current passing through an inductor. When current begins to flow through the inductor, magnetic lines of force are generated. The energy used to make this magnetic field comes from the voltage source. As magnetic lines of force are developed around each coil, they can be considered moving lines of magnetic force (just as waves radiate or move out from the disturbance caused when a pebble is dropped into a pool of water). As discussed previously, if moving magnetic lines of force cut across a conductor, a current is induced. Fig. 8-3 illustrates that current in one half of the looped wire will induce a current flow in the other half, because moving magnetic lines of force are cutting across the adjacent conducting wires. However, note that this induced current or EMF (which causes current to flow) opposes the direction of current flow from the voltage source. Or it can be said that the induced EMF is a counter EMF, that is, opposing the EMF of the source.

In a direct current circuit, the only other time the magnetic lines of force move

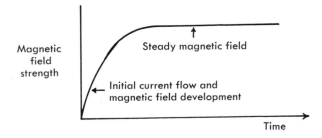

Fig. 8-4. Development of magnetic field around current-carrying conductor in dc circuit.

is when the current stops and the magnetic field collapses. When the field collapses a counter EMF is momentarily established that causes a brief counter EMF or "kick back" current in the circuit.

After the initial generation of the magnetic field around the looped conductors of an inductor in a dc circuit, there is no effect exerted on direct current flow. It is important to remember that once the lines of magnetic force are stationary, they cannot cut across a conductor. Therefore, a current or EMF cannot be induced. Thus, in a dc circuit, an inductor is considered to be essentially a straight wire, exerting only the effect of the resistance offered by that wire. Why not consider the effects exerted by the initial current flow and the stopping of current flow? The answer is that these effects are only momentarily exerted and do not exist during the continual operation of the circuit. Therefore, for all practical purposes, the effect of a counter EMF exerted by a coil does not exist in a dc circuit. Fig. 8-4 shows the development of a magnetic field around a conductor passing a dc current.

Direct current is essentially unaffected by an inductor. But it is given careful consideration in this chapter to express as simply as possible the development of a counter EMF in an inductor. Once this concept is understood, the effect of an inductor on alternating current can be more easily appreciated.

INDUCTOR IN AN AC CIRCUIT

An inductor exerts an impedance to alternating current that is directly proportional to the frequency of the alternating current passing through the inductor. When an alternating current is passed through an inductor, the magnetic field produced varies at the same rate and in proportion to the magnitude of the current. The result is a constantly moving magnetic field. As the current increases, the magnetic lines of force radiate out from the conductor, and as the current decreases, the magnetic lines of force begin to collapse. This moving or "pulsating magnetic field" cuts across the adjacent turns of the coil, thus producing a back or counter EMF. The faster the magnetic field "pulsates," the greater the counter EMF induced. Therefore, with increased frequency of an alternating current there is developed a greater counter EMF or hindrance to current flow. Impedance increases as frequency increases.

Summarized here is the development of a counter EMF in an inductor. An important characteristic of alternating current is that voltage and current amplitude are continually changing. As the current begins to increase through the inductor, the magnetic lines of flux expand around each turn of the inductor. The expanding field cuts through the adjacent turns of the inductor, which results in a current being induced in those adjacent turns. The induced current flows in the opposite direction to the original current. This phenomenon is expressed in Lenz's law, which states: "When a current is induced in a coil as a result of any variation in the magnetic field surrounding the coil, the induced current is in such a direction as to oppose the current change that produced the magnetic variation."

INDUCTANCE AND INDUCTIVE REACTANCE

Induction of one volt resulting from a current variation of one ampere per second equals one *henry* (H). Other units of inductance are the millihenry (mH), one thousandth of a henry, and the microhenry (μH), one millionth of a henry.

The inductance of an inductor is determined by the characteristics of its construction, including number and diameter of turns, system of winding, coil length-diameter ratio, and core material. The way a coil is constructed depends upon the effect it is meant to produce in the circuit. The core material contained within the center or core of the inductor may be air or a magnetic material such as iron. Air-core inductors are made by winding wire on a nonmagnetic material to serve as a support or by using wire sufficiently heavy to be self-supporting. A magnetic core increases the inductance of an inductor by concentrating the magnetic field within the coil. An inductor having a movable iron core is a variable inductor, the inductance of which can be varied by adjusting the length of the iron core inside the coil.

Inductance (L) is the property that opposes change in current flow. Inductive reactance (X_L) is the impedance or effective resistance offered by an inductor to alternating current. Its unit of measurement is the ohm. The formula used to calculate inductive reactance is:

$$X_L = 2\pi fL$$

where:

X_L = Inductive reactance in ohms
π = A constant (3.14)
f = Frequency of applied voltage in hertz
L = Inductance in henrys

Note that once a fixed inductor is constructed, the frequency of the applied voltage is the only variable capable of changing the inductive reactance.

The information derived from the above formula is better appreciated when an ac frequency change is related to the resulting change in the inductive reactance.

What would the inductive reactance be for a 200 mH inductor if applied across it is a 120 Vac signal having a frequency of:

1. 50 Hz
2. 100 Hz
3. 200 Hz

Solutions:

$$X_L = 2\pi fL$$

1. $X_L = (2)(3.14)(50 \text{ Hz})(0.2 \text{ H}) = 62.8 \ \Omega$
2. $X_L = (2)(3.14)(100 \text{ Hz})(0.2 \text{ H}) = 125.6 \ \Omega$
3. $X_L = (2)(3.14)(200 \text{ Hz})(0.2 \text{ H}) = 251.2 \ \Omega$

As the frequency increases, the inductive reactance increases. This is opposite to the effect frequency has on capacitive reactance, in which an increase in frequency decreases the capacitive reactance.

In a purely inductive circuit, inductive reactance (X_L) can be substituted for impedance (Z) so that, for ac circuits, Ohm's law is changed from $Z = E/I$ to $X_L = E/I$.

PHASE RELATIONSHIP IN AN INDUCTOR

Current and voltage are in phase when an ac voltage is applied across a resistor. In other words, maximum voltage causes maximum current, and minimum voltage causes minimum current. Thus, a direct phase relationship exists between voltage and current (Fig. 8-5).

Review the phase relationship of voltage and current when an ac voltage is applied across a capacitor. Maximum current flows first; then as the voltage increases across the capacitor, the current decreases. In this case current leads voltage. The phase difference has been determined to be 90°. The current leads the voltage by 90° in a capacitive circuit.

In an inductive circuit, when an alternating current is applied across an inductor, the voltage leads the current by 90°. As a voltage is applied to the inductor, a current starts to flow, causing the formation of a magnetic field that induces a counter EMF to oppose the increase of current flow. This hindrance to current flow delays changes in current 90° behind changes in voltage (Fig. 8-6).

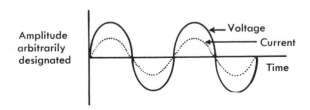

Fig. 8-5. Phase relationship of ac voltage and current across a resistor.

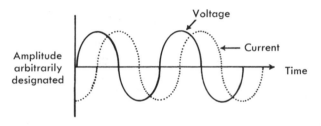

Fig. 8-6. Phase relationship of ac voltage and current across an inductor.

INDUCTORS IN SERIES, PARALLEL, AND SERIES-PARALLEL

Inductors in proximity in a circuit may impose the effects of their magnetic fields upon each other. This is usually undesirable. Circuits may not perform effectively those functions for which they were designed if interfering, unpredictable forces are generated. Thus, the rules for determining the total effective inductive reactance of inductors connected in series, parallel, or series-parallel are applicable only if the inductors' magnetic fields cannot act upon each other. The total effective inductance of inductors connected in series is calculated with this equation: $L_{total} = L_1 + L_2 + L_3 \ldots L_n$. The total effective inductance of inductors connected in parallel can be calculated with the equation: $1/L_{total} = 1/L_1 + 1/L_2 + 1/L_3 \ldots 1/L_n$.

RESISTANCE AND IMPEDANCE

The total effective impedance exerted by an inductor and a resistor connected in series is determined by using this equation: $Z = \sqrt{R^2 + X_L^2}$. The total effective impedance exerted by an inductor and resistor connected in parallel can be determined by using the equation: $Z = (R)(X_L)/\sqrt{R^2 + X_L^2}$.

Table 1. A summary comparison of resistors, capacitors, and inductors in dc and ac circuits

Circuit	Property	Resistor	Capacitor	Inductor
dc	Resistance	Resistance (R) Unit = ohm R = E/I	Infinite resistance	Negligible resistance
ac	Impedance	Impedance (Z) Unit = ohm Z = E/I	Capacitive reactance (X_C) Unit = ohm $X_C = 1/2\pi fC$	Inductive reactance (X_L) Unit = ohm $X_L = 2\pi fL$
ac	Phase relationship between voltage and current	In phase	Current leads voltage by 90°	Voltage leads current by 90°

INSTRUCTIONAL ACTIVITIES

1. Display different types of inductors. Expose the construction of inoperable inductors.
2. Students are to identify inductors in circuits of commonly used instruments.
3. Demonstrate with an ammeter that a dc current through an inductor is initially decreased with the expansion of the magnetic field and is increased with the collapse of the magnetic field.
4. Demonstrate that a current is induced by a magnetic field cutting across a conductor. Place two insulated straight wires next to each other. Pass a current through the first

wire while monitoring with a very sensitive ammeter (microampere range) the current in the second wire.

Current pulses should be detected in the second wire the instant the voltage is applied across the first wire and the instant the voltage is removed from the first wire. The current pulses observed in the second wire will flow in the direction opposite to the current in the first wire.

PRACTICE PROBLEMS and STUDY QUESTIONS

1. Calculate the impedance of a 150 mH inductor in a circuit to which is applied 115 Vac at a frequency of:
   a. 4000 Hz
   b. 2000 Hz
   c. 200 Hz
   d. 20 Hz
2. Calculate total effective inductance, total effective impedance, and current in a 220 Vac, 60 Hz, circuit in which two inductors ($L_1 = 600$ mH and $L_2 = 300$ mH) are connected in:
   a. Series
   b. Parallel
3.

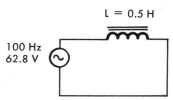

What is the current in the circuit above?
4. For each of the following three circuits calculate:
   a. Total effective impedance
   b. Current

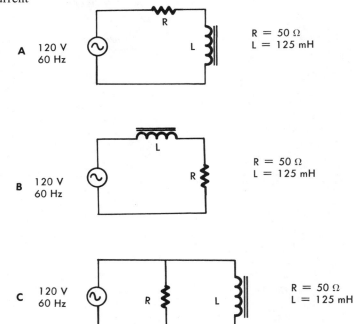

5. Will impedance be increased, decreased, or unchanged in each of the following cases:
   a. Decreasing the frequency of ac passing through an inductor
   b. Doubling the dc voltage passing through a coil
   c. Increasing the ac frequency passing through a capacitor
   d. Decreasing the amplitude of ac passing through a coil
   e. Increasing the frequency of ac passing through a resistor
6. Match the following terms and definitions, using each lettered answer only once:

    ___(1) Opposition to a change in current   A. Inductance
          flow with development of back EMF   B. Current
    ___(2) Rate of movement of a charge   C. Resistance
          through a conductor   D. Power
    ___(3) Causes electrons to move through   E. Inductive reactance
          a conductor   F. Capacitance
    ___(4) Impedance offered by a coil to ac   G. Electromotive force
    ___(5) Ability of capacitors to store   H. Capacitive reactance
          electrical charge   I. Infinite resistance
    ___(6) Volts/amperes
    ___(7) Resistance of a capacitor to dc
    ___(8) Work done when electrons move
          through a resistance
    ___(9) Resistance of a capacitor to ac

7. List the unit of measure for each of the following:
   a. Inductance
   b. Current
   c. Resistance
   d. Power
   e. Inductive reactance
   f. Capacitance
   g. Electromotive force
   h. Capacitive reactance
8. Match each unit of measure with its definition, using each lettered answer only once:

    ___(1) Cumulative charge of 6.24×10^{18} A. Coulomb
          electrons   B. Volt
    ___(2) Force required to move one coulomb   C. Ampere
          per second through a resistance of   D. Ohm
          one ohm   E. Henry
    ___(3) The capacity to store one coulomb   F. Farad
          of electrical energy when one volt
          is applied to two parallel plates
          separated by a dielectric
    ___(4) When a current change of one
          ampere per second causes a back
          EMF of one volt in a coiled wire
    ___(5) A value of resistance through which
          one volt maintains a current of one
          ampere
    ___(6) One coulomb passing a point in a
          circuit every second

ANSWERS

1. a. 3.768 kΩ
   b. 1.884 kΩ
   c. 188.4 Ω
   d. 18.84 Ω
2. a. L_T = 900 mH; X_L = 339.12 Ω; I = 648.7 mA.
   b. L_T = 0.2 H; X_L = 75.36 Ω; I = 2.92 A
3. 200 mA
4. Fig. *A*   a. Z = 4.718 kΩ   b. I = 25.43 mA
   Fig. *B*   a. Z = 4.718 kΩ   b. I = 25.43 mA
   Fig. *C*   a. Z = 34.28 Ω   b. I = 3.5 A
5. a. Decreased
   b. Unchanged
   c. Decreased
   d. Unchanged
   e. Unchanged

6. (1) A   7. a. Henry   8. (1) A
   (2) B   b. Ampere   (2) B
   (3) G   c. Ohm   (3) F
   (4) E   d. Watt   (4) E
   (5) F   e. Ohm   (5) D
   (6) C   f. Farad   (6) C
   (7) I   g. Volt
   (8) D   h. Ohm
   (9) H

APPROACH TO SOLVING PROBLEMS

1. a. X_L = $2\pi fL$ = (2)(3.14)(4000 Hz)(0.15 H) = 3.768 kΩ
   b. X_L = $2\pi fL$ = (2)(3.14)(2000 Hz)(0.15 H) = 1.884 kΩ
   c. X_L = $2\pi fL$ = (2)(3.14)(200 Hz)(0.15 H) = 188.4 Ω
   d. X_L = $2\pi fL$ = (2)(3.14)(20 Hz)(0.15 H) = 18.84 Ω
2. a. L_T = L_1 + L_2 = 600 mH + 300 mH = 900 mH
      X_L = $2\pi fL$ = (2)(3.14)(60 Hz)(0.9 H) = 339.12 Ω
      I = E/X_L = 220 V/339.12 Ω = 648.7 mA
   b. L_T = $(L_1)(L_2)/(L_1)$ + (L_2) = 0.18/0.9 = 0.2 H
      X_L = $2\pi fL$ = (2)(3.14)(60 Hz)(0.2 H) = 75.36 Ω
      I = E/X_L = 220 V/75.36 Ω = 2.92 A
3. X_L = $2\pi fL$ = (2)(3.14)(100 Hz)(0.5 H) = 314 Ω
   I = E/X_L = 62.8 V/ 314 Ω = 200 mA
4. Fig. *A*   a. X_L = $2\pi fL$ = (2)(3.14)(60 Hz)(0.125 H) = 47.1 Ω
      Z = R^2 + X_L^2 = 50^2 + 47.1^2 = 2.5 kΩ + 2.218 kΩ = 4.718 kΩ
      b.   I = E/X_L = 120 V/4.718 kΩ = 25.43 mA
   Fig. *B*   a. X_L = $2\pi fL$ = (2)(3.14)(60 Hz)(0.125 H) = 47.1 Ω
      Z = R^2 + X_L^2 = 50^2 + 47.1^2 = 2.5 kΩ + 2.218 kΩ = 4.718 kΩ
      b.   I = E/X_L = 120 V/4.718 kΩ = 25.43 mA
   Fig. *C*   a. X_L = $2\pi fL$ = (2)(3.14)(60 Hz)(0.125) = 47.1 Ω
      Z = $(R)(X_L)/\sqrt{R^2 + X_L^2}$ = 2355 Ω/$\sqrt{4718}$ = 2355/68.69 = 34.28 Ω
      b.   I = E/X_L = 120 V/34.28 Ω = 3.5 A

CHAPTER 9

TRANSFORMERS

Transformers are extensively used in electronic instruments. They commonly function to change the level of input voltage to meet voltage level requirements of various circuits in an instrument. The input ac voltage applied across a transformer may be decreased or increased or may remain unchanged. Transformers may also serve to block unwanted direct current from passing from one circuit to another.

INDUCTION OF CURRENT

When an alternating current passes through a coil, the changing current causes a changing magnetic field. The expanding and collapsing of a magnetic field around a coiled, ac current-carrying wire results in the generation of a back EMF. This inductance of a back EMF in a coil is called self-inductance.

There is another type of current induction that plays an important role in most analytical instruments. This is the induction of a current in one coil by the current flowing in another separate coil. Two separate coils in parallel orientation and in proximity to each other are the arrangement required for this type of current induction. When ac current is passed through one of the coils (primary coil) but not through the other, a current can be measured in both coils. The coil not attached to a potential (secondary coil) has had a current induced in it by the constantly changing magnetic field generated by the alternating current in the first coil (Fig. 9-1).

Note that if a dc current were passed through the primary coil, a constant

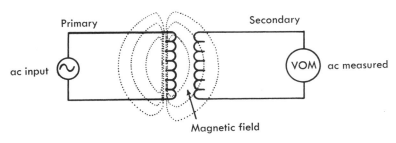

Primary   Secondary

ac input   VOM   ac measured

Magnetic field

Fig. 9-1. Current induction.

current would not be induced in the secondary coil. A current pulse in the secondary coil could be measured only during two specific times — one pulse with the initiation of dc current flow and the other with its termination. Current is induced at these two particular times because only during initiation and termination of dc current flow is there a change in the magnetic field — that is, expansion and collapse, respectively.

TRANSFORMER CONSTRUCTION

The phenomenon of current induction in one coil by an ac current in another coil is employed in a transformer. The construction of a transformer allows for maximum power transfer from one coil to the other. Two factors to be considered are the proximity of the coils and the concentration of the magnetic field. The closer the coils, the greater the effectiveness of current induction. Therefore, the insulated wires can be wound over each other around a central core. A central and peripheral iron core is used to concentrate the magnetic field about the coils because current induction is directly related to the strength of the magnetic field (Fig. 9-2).

Symbolic representations of transformers are:

Air-core: Iron-core:

TRANSFORMER ACTION

Induction of current is accompanied by induction of voltage and dissipation of power. These three factors are inseparable. Voltage is the electrical factor most frequently used to describe induced energy because the input voltage on the primary coil induces a voltage in the secondary coil simultaneously with current induction.

The ac voltage induced in the secondary coil is 180° out of phase with the ac voltage across the primary coil. The positive half of an input sine wave generates magnetic lines of force that cut across the secondary coil in a direction opposite to the direction they are generated from the primary. Therefore, when the input

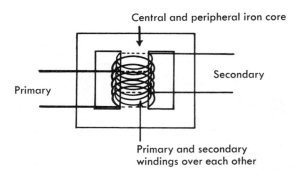

Fig. 9-2. Iron-core transformer.

voltage is positive the voltage across the secondary is negative, and when the input voltage is negative the secondary voltage is positive (Fig. 9-3).

An equation used to calculate the voltage induced in the secondary coil by the primary coil is:

$$E_s/E_p = N_s/N_p$$

where:

E_s = Voltage in secondary coil
E_p = Voltage in primary coil
N_s = Number of turns in secondary coil
N_p = Number of turns in primary coil

As seen in the equation, the voltage induced is directly related to the number of turns in the coils. If there are more turns in the secondary coil than in the primary, the magnetic field of the primary obviously will cut across more conducting wires in the secondary, therefore inducing a larger voltage. This type of transformer is called a "step-up" transformer (Fig. 9-4). On the other hand, if there are fewer turns in the secondary coil than in the primary coil, the transformer is a "step-down" transformer (Fig. 9-5).

In another type of transformer, there are multiple secondary windings to provide several levels of induced voltages (Fig. 9-6).

The equation above is applied in the following sample problems:

1. What voltage is induced in a secondary coil of 150 turns if 120 Vac is applied across the primary of 100 turns? (Step-up transformer)

Solution:

$$E_s/E_p = N_s/N_p$$
$$E_s/120 \text{ Vac} = 150/100$$
$$E_s = 18000/100 = 180 \text{ Vac}$$

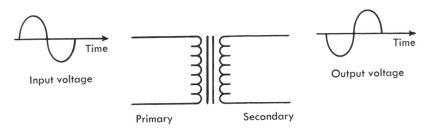

Fig. 9-3. Transformer action.

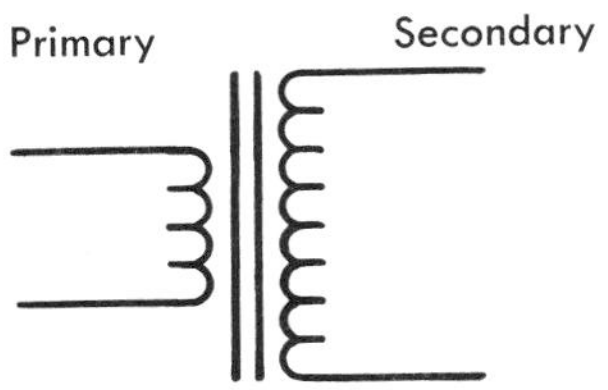

Fig. 9-4. Step-up transformer.

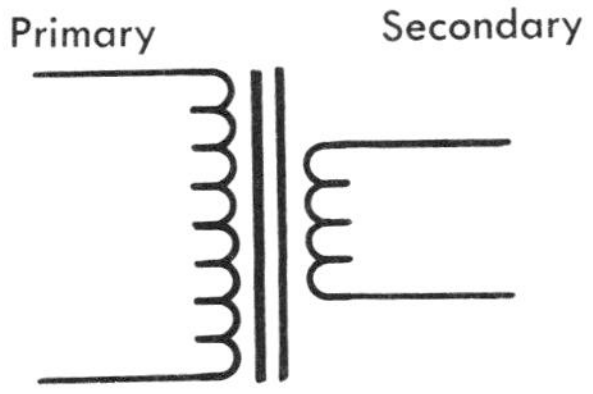

Fig. 9-5. Step-down transformer.

Primary   Secondary

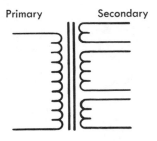

Fig. 9-6. Transformer with multiple secondary windings.

2. What voltage is induced in a secondary coil of 75 turns if 120 Vac is applied across the primary of 100 turns? (Step-down transformer)

Solution:

$$E_s/E_p = N_s/N_p$$
$$E_s/120 \text{ Vac} = 75/100$$
$$E_s = 9000/100 = 90 \text{ Vac}$$

In both step-up and step-down transformers it appears that voltage is magically magnified or diminished and that the law of conservation of energy is ignored. Not true! The energy transferred between the primary and secondary coils is power. The power in the primary coil equals the power in the secondary if the transformer is 100% efficient. Consider this ideal case:

$$P_p = P_s$$

Power is the product of current and voltage. Therefore:

$$I_p \times E_p = I_2 \times E_s$$

Thus, if voltage is stepped up, the current is proportionately stepped down, and if the voltage is stepped down, the current is stepped up. To demonstrate this concept, consider these problems:

In each of the previous problems, 1 and 2, if the power in the primary were 60 W, what would be the current in the primary and in the secondary?

$$I_s = 60 \text{ W}/180 \text{ V} = 0.333 \text{ A}$$
(Note that in the secondary coil the voltage increased and the current decreased.)

2. Current in the primary $I_p = P_p/E_p$
$$I_p = 60 \text{ W}/120 \text{ V} = 0.5 \text{ A}$$
    Current in the secondary $I_s = P_s/E_s$
$$I_s = 60 \text{ W}/90 \text{ V} = 0.667 \text{ A}$$
(Note that in the secondary coil the current increased and the voltage decreased.)

Another useful application of transformers is the isolation of certain ac circuits and/or components from unwanted direct current. As discussed earlier, direct current is unable to induce a current. Therefore, while alternating current will be transmitted through a transformer, direct current will be blocked.

INSTRUCTIONAL ACTIVITIES

1. Display a transformer both in a circuit and not in a circuit.
2. Connect an oscilloscope or VOM across the secondary side of a transformer.
   a. Apply a dc input voltage across the primary side of the transformer, and request that the students note their observations.
      (1) A voltage pulse across the secondary is detected with the initial application of dc voltage to the primary.
      (2) With constant application of dc voltage to the primary, no voltage is detected across the secondary.
      (3) A voltage pulse across the secondary is detected with the termination of the application of dc voltage to the primary.
   b. Apply an ac input voltage across the primary side of the transformer, and request that the students note their observations.
      (1) With constant application of ac voltage to primary, an ac voltage is detected across the secondary.
      (2) Using the value of input voltage and the value of voltage in the secondary, students can classify the transformer as step-up or step-down.
3. If a dual channel oscilloscope is available, connect one channel across the primary and the other across the secondary of a transformer. Apply an ac input voltage across the primary, and request that the students note their observations.
   a. A phase shift of 180° between primary and secondary voltages is observed.
   b. The frequency of the voltage is unaffected by transformer action.
   c. The values of voltages in the primary and the secondary can be used to classify the transformer as step-up or step-down.
4. Given a VOM and a transformer (for example, a 6.3 V transformer) not connected in a circuit, students are to classify the transformer as either step-up or step-down. Resistance of the primary and the secondary windings is directly related to the number of windings, since the resistance is directly related to the length of the wire. Therefore, if the primary side has a higher resistance than the secondary, the transformer is a step-down transformer. The opposite is true of a step-up transformer.

PRACTICE PROBLEMS and STUDY QUESTIONS

1. Given a transformer with:
   Turns in the primary = 80
   Resistance of primary coil = 100 Ω
   Resistance of secondary coil = 140 Ω
   Power dissipated = 60 W
   Input voltage = 120 Vac

   Determine:
   a. Type of transformer (step-up or step-down)
   b. Number of turns in the secondary coil
   c. Voltage induced in the secondary coil
   d. Current in the primary coil
   e. Current in the secondary coil
2. The primary side of a transformer has 25 turns and 125 Vac applied across it. The secondary side of this transformer has 50 turns and power of 100 W.
   a. What is the induced voltage in the secondary coil?
   b. What is the current in the secondary coil?
   c. What is the current in the primary coil?

3. In the transformer shown below, 6 watts is dissipated in the primary and secondary coils. Calculate the voltage and the current for each of the three secondary coils: a, b, and c.

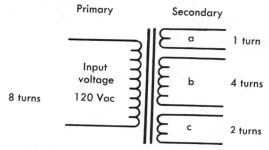

ANSWERS
1. a. Step-up
   b. 112
   c. 168 Vac
   d. 0.67 A
   e. 0.48 A
2. a. 250 Vac
   b. 0.4 A
   c. 0.8 A
3. a: 15 Vac and 0.4 A
   b: 60 Vac and 0.1 A
   c: 30 Vac and 0.2 A

APPROACH TO SOLVING PROBLEMS
1. b. (80 turns)(140/100) = 112
   c. (120 Vac)(140/100) = 168 Vac
   d. I_p = 80 W/120 Vac = 0.67 A
   e. I_s = 80 W/168 Vac = 0.48 A
2. a. $E_s/E_p = N_s/N_p$
   $E_s/125$ Vac = 50/25
   E_s = 250 Vac
   b. $I_s = P_s/E_s$ = 100 W/250 Vac = 0.4 A
   c. $I_p = P_p/E_p$ = 100 W/125 Vac = 0.8 A
3. Voltage
   a: $E_s/E_p = N_s/N_p$; $E_s/120$ Vac = 1/8; E_s = 120 Vac/8 = 15 Vac
   b: $E_s/E_p = N_s/N_p$; $E_s/120$ Vac = 4/8; E_s = 480 Vac/8 = 60 Vac
   c: $E_s/E_p = N_s/N_p$; $E_s/120$ Vac = 2/8; E_s = 240 Vac/8 = 30 Vac
   Current
   a: $I_s = P_s/E_s$ = 6 W/15 Vac = 0.4 A
   b: $I_s = P_s/E_s$ = 6 W/60 Vac = 0.1 A
   c: $I_s = P_s/E_s$ = 6 W/30 Vac = 0.2 A

CHAPTER 10

DIODES

Diodes are electronic components with a simple design not representative of their importance. The diode (*di* meaning two and *ode* from electrode) is a two-electrode unit that plays a major role in rectification of alternating current to direct current. There are two types of diodes—vacuum tube and semiconductor. An examination of the construction and operation of each type will be followed by a discussion of diode applications.

VACUUM TUBE DIODE

Vacuum tubes are disappearing from electronic circuits and being replaced by semiconductors. However, a consideration of vacuum tube principles of operation will contribute to the understanding of rectification and, later, amplification. The operational principles of vacuum tubes are conceptually clear and therefore easily understood. These principles can be used to aid in understanding semiconductor operational principles.

The function of vacuum tubes is based upon two fundamental principles—thermionic emission and attraction and repulsion of unlike and like charges, respectively. Thermionic emission is the release of electrons caused by an increased temperature of particular metals. The rise in temperature imparts enough energy to some electrons to result in their liberation from the heated metal. The freed electrons collect at the surface of the metal, forming an electron cloud (Fig. 10-1).

A diode consists of two electrodes and a heater, all of which are encased within an evacuated glass envelope. The electrodes are the cathode and the plate. The cathode is the electrode that is heated and from which electrons are emitted. Tungsten is commonly used for the cathode. The plate is the collector of emitted electrons.

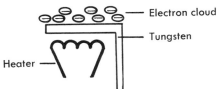

Fig. 10-1. Thermionic emission.

The heater supplies heat to the cathode. The cathode can be directly or indirectly heated (Fig. 10-2). Since the heater element plays an indirect role in the function of the diode, it is frequently not shown in schematic representations of vacuum tube diodes. Regardless of whether the heater element is shown, its presence in a vacuum tube diode is understood.

Operation of a vacuum tube diode depends upon the voltage at each of the two electrodes — cathode and plate. When the plate is positive in relation to the cathode, the diode is said to be "forward biased." Electrons are attracted to the plate, and a current flows. In a "reverse-biased" diode, the plate is negative with respect to the cathode. A current will not pass through this diode, since the negative charges on the plate and on the cathode will repel each other. A forward-biased diode is said to be conducting, and a reverse-biased diode is said to be nonconducting (Fig. 10-3).

Forward- and reverse-biased vacuum tube diodes in simple circuits are shown in Fig. 10-4. When the battery is connected with the negative side to the cathode and the positive side to the plate, the forward-biased diode conducts and a current flows in the circuit. The electrons emitted from the cathode and attracted to the positive side of the battery are replenished by the electrons from the negative side of the battery, and a constant current flows in the circuit (Fig. 10-4, *A*). When the battery is connected with the positive side to the cathode and the negative side to the plate, the reverse-biased diode does not conduct. The electrons emitted from the cathode are repelled by the negative charge on the plate. Since no current can pass through the diode, the circuit is not complete and current will not flow (Fig. 10-4, *B*).

Voltage and current in the anode circuit of the vacuum tube diode are designated plate voltage (E_p) and plate current (I_p), respectively. Since there is a potential difference between the cathode and the plate in a conducting diode, there is a voltage drop across the diode. According to Ohm's law, a voltage drop occurs across a resistance. The resistance of a vacuum tube diode is called plate resistance (R_p) and is calculated:

$$R_p = E_p/I_p$$

SEMICONDUCTOR DIODES

A semiconductor electronic component is also called a solid-state device. Thus the names "semiconductor diode" and "solid-state diode" are interchangeable. Semiconductor and vacuum tube diodes have similar circuit applications but different operational principles.

The operation of a semiconductor diode is based upon its crystalline structure and composition. As discussed earlier, a conductor is a material whose atoms contain loosely bound electrons, and an insulator is composed of atoms that bind their electrons very tightly. Some pure crystalline substances, such as silicon and germanium, are semiconductors. The conductivity of semiconductors is between that of insulators and conductors, depending upon the temperature of the crystal.

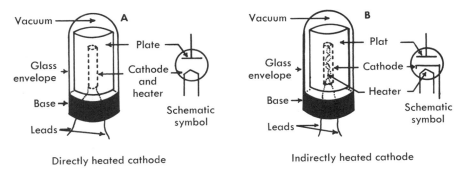

Directly heated cathode   Indirectly heated cathode

Fig. 10-2. Arrangement of elements in vacuum tube diode.

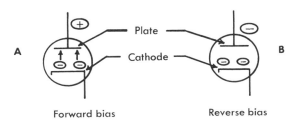

Forward bias   Reverse bias

Fig. 10-3. Vacuum tube diode bias.

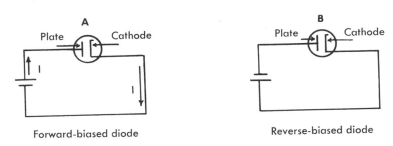

Forward-biased diode   Reverse-biased diode

Fig. 10-4. Vacuum tube diode in circuit.

Conductivity increases with increase in temperature. The crystalline structure of a pure germanium crystal is shown in Fig. 10-5.

The pure crystal can be changed to enhance conductivity by adding a specific impurity. The addition of the impurity is called "doping." The impurity must have a structure compatable with the crystalline structure of the pure crystal to allow for its incorporation into the crystal. Depending upon whether the doping element is a donor or acceptor impurity, the crystal may have an excess or deficit of loosely bound electrons. A donor impurity is a pentavalent element, for example, arsenic, antimony, or phosphorus, that provides one free electron per atom incorporated. The excess electrons are not held in covalent bonds and therefore are free to move within the crystal. An acceptor impurity is a trivalent

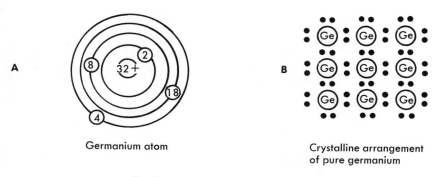

Germanium atom

Crystalline arrangement
of pure germanium

Fig. 10-5. Germanium atom and crystalline form.

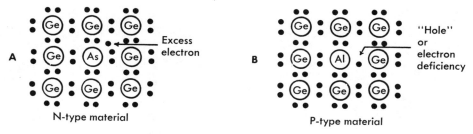

Excess
electron

"Hole"
or
electron
deficiency

N-type material

P-type material

Fig. 10-6. Impurity semiconductor crystals.

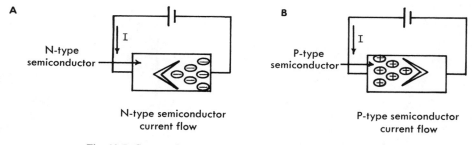

N-type
semiconductor

P-type
semiconductor

N-type semiconductor
current flow

P-type semiconductor
current flow

Fig. 10-7. Current flow through N-type and P-type semiconductors.

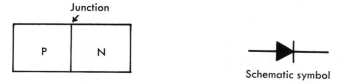

Junction

P   N

Schematic symbol

Fig. 10-8. P-N junction diode.

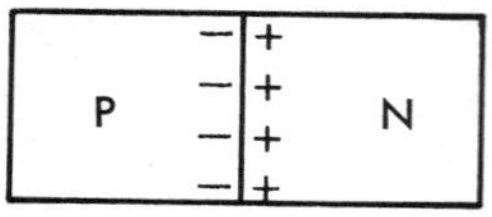

P   N

Fig. 10-9. Potential barrier between P-type and N-type semiconductors in semiconductor diode.

element, such as aluminum, gallium, or boron. The acceptor impurity provides the pure crystal with an electron deficit of one electron per atom of impurity incorporated into the crystal. This electron deficit is called a "hole." Conceptually, a hole can be thought of as a positive charge.

A pure crystal doped with a pentavalent or trivalent impurity is called an extrinsic or impurity semiconductor. Impurity semiconductors are of two types, N-type and P-type. The N-type has excess electrons known as negative carriers resulting from a donor impurity (Fig. 10-6, *A*). An acceptor impurity supplies a pure crystal with excess holes known as positive carriers, thus producing a P-type semiconductor (Fig. 10-6, *B*). The addition of an impurity to a pure crystal does not give the crystal a net charge. The neutrality of the crystal is maintained, since the added atoms have an equal number of electrons and protons. The terms "electron excess" and "electron deficit" refer to the availability of or lack of mobile electrons.

When a potential is placed across an N-type or P-type semiconductor, each conducts a current. However, the method of current conduction differs in each type. A potential applied across an N-type semiconductor causes current to flow because of the negative carriers (Fig. 10-7, *A*). Current flow through a P-type semiconductor results from the apparent movement of positive carriers (holes) through the semiconductor (Fig. 10-7, *B*).

P-type and N-type semiconductor materials are used to construct a semiconductor diode, also referred to as a P-N junction diode. The P-N junction diode is made by chemically fusing a P-type crystal and an N-type crystal (Fig. 10-8). After the two materials are fused, a few majority carriers of each diffuse across the interface. The negative carriers moving into the proximal P-type crystal and the positive carriers moving into the adjacent N-type crystal result in a small potential being formed across the junction. This potential, called a potential gradient or potential barrier, impedes further charge diffusion across the junction (Fig. 10-9).

Current can be caused to flow across a P-N junction if an external potential greater than the potential barrier biases the P-N junction in a forward direction. The potential across the semiconductor diode is referred to as "bias." The bias can be forward or reverse. Fig. 10-10, *A*, represents a circuit in which a current is conducted through a forward-biased semiconductor. The positive terminal of the battery is connected to the P-type semiconductor and the negative terminal to the N-type semiconductor. The positive and negative carriers are repelled by the battery's positive and negative charges, respectively. The holes and the electrons cross the barrier potential and recombine. Conceptually, the electrons and holes meet at the junction and neutralize each other. The net result is conventional current flow from the positive terminal to the negative terminal.

A semiconductor connected in a circuit, negative potential to P-type and positive potential to N-type semiconductor, is reverse biased (Fig. 10-10, *B*). The positive carriers in the P-type semiconductor are attracted to the negative potential, and the negative carriers are attracted to the positive potential. Since both types of carrier charges move away from the P-N junction, no current is con-

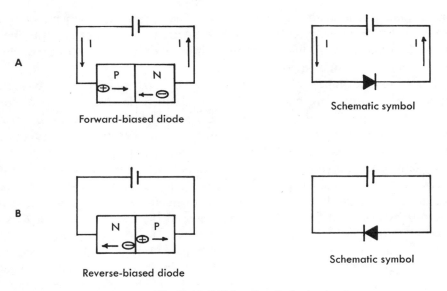

A Forward-biased diode

Schematic symbol

B Reverse-biased diode

Schematic symbol

Fig. 10-10. P-N junction diodes in circuit.

ducted through the diode. Conceptually, the semiconductor material at the junction becomes a good insulator.

If the voltage rating of a particular semiconductor diode is exceeded, the diode can be ruined. If an excess potential is placed across a reverse-biased semiconductor diode, an avalanche current results as electrons are forced from valence bonds. An avalanche current destroys the integrity of the P-N junction in conventional semiconductor diodes. However, there is a class of semiconductor diodes called zener diodes (symbol: ———), which are designed to conduct only avalanche current. Zener diodes function at the reverse breakdown point and are used for regulation of voltage, although this is not their primary application. A zener diode is strategically placed in a circuit at a point where voltage level must not exceed a predetermined level. When that level is exceeded, the excess voltage is dropped through the zener diode with avalanche current flow.

DIODE APPLICATIONS

As mentioned above, specifically designed semiconductor diodes are used for voltage regulation. However, the primary function of diodes is to rectify alternating current to direct current. Both vacuum tube and semiconductor diodes are unidirectional current devices, that is, allowing current to flow in only one direction. Each, therefore, is capable of converting ac voltage to dc voltage. Semiconductor diodes will be used in circuit diagrams for demonstrating rectification. However, in each case the semiconductor diode could be replaced with a vacuum tube diode (See Fig. 10-11. Note that the output signal is monitored with an oscilloscope also called a cathode ray tube, abbreviated CRT.)

Rectification is shown in Fig. 10-12. During the positive half-cycle of the input ac signal at the transformer's secondary winding, the diode is forward biased. The

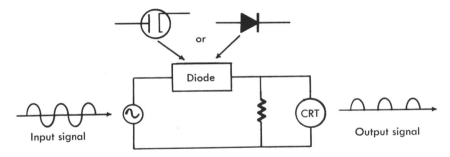

Fig. 10-11. Rectification.

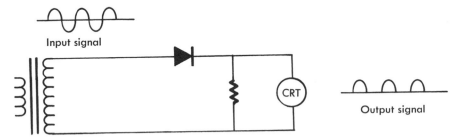

Fig. 10-12. Half-wave rectifier.

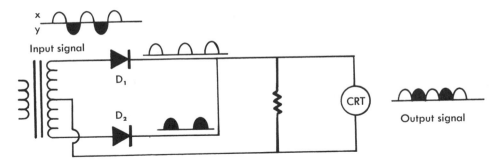

Fig. 10-13. Full-wave rectifier.

forward-biased diode conducts, and an output voltage results. When the half-cycle of the input signal is negative, the diode is reverse biased, no current is conducted, and there is no output voltage. With each full cycle of input ac voltage, only the positive half of the cycle is conducted through the diode. This is half-wave rectification.

Fig. 10-13 shows a circuit containing two diodes functioning as a full-wave rectifier. During half-cycle X, D_1 is forward biased and conducts, while D_2 is reverse biased and does not conduct. The opposite is true during half-cycle Y. D_2 is forward biased and conducts, while reverse-biased D_1 does not. The output of a full-wave rectifier contains the voltage of both the half-cycles of the input ac voltage. Since the output voltage does not change polarity, it is dc voltage. Thus ac voltage has been changed to dc voltage by the action of diodes.

INSTRUCTIONAL ACTIVITIES

1. Display two types of diodes:
   a. Vacuum tube diode
   b. Semiconductor diode
2. Demonstrate unidirectional current passing capability of the diode. Using a battery, a resistor, a diode, and an ammeter, build the circuits shown below.

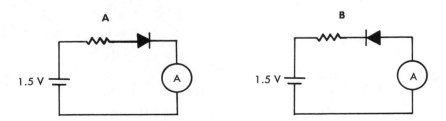

The diode in circuit *A* is forward biased; therefore, current flow will be indicated by the ammeter. The diode in circuit *B* is reverse biased; therefore, no current will be registered on the ammeter.

3. Demonstrate half-wave and full-wave rectification. Using a transformer with a center tap, diodes, a resistor, and an oscilloscope, build the following circuits.

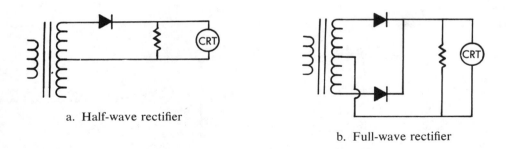

a. Half-wave rectifier

b. Full-wave rectifier

The output signals of each circuit will be seen on the oscilloscope.

PRACTICE PROBLEMS and STUDY QUESTIONS

1. What is the plate resistance of a vacuum tube diode if the plate voltage is 2 V and the plate current is 10 mA?
2. Are the diodes in the following circuits forward or reverse biased?

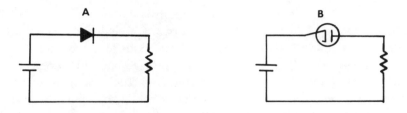

3. Draw the output voltage signals shown on the CRT in each of the following circuits.

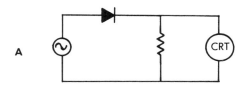

A

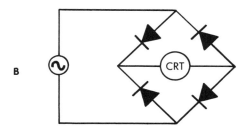

B

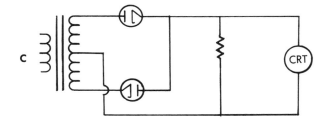

C

ANSWERS

1. 200 Ω
2. A. Forward biased
   B. Reverse biased
3.
   A.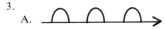

   B. ⌢⌢⌢⌢⌢ →

   C. ⌢ ⌢ ⌢ →

APPROACH TO SOLVING PROBLEMS

1. $R_p = E_p/I_p = 2$ V$/0.01$ A $= 200$ Ω

Electronic functional units of analytical instruments

Basic principles of electronics and descriptive detail about components have been presented in earlier sections. Isolated concepts and facts, however, carry little relevance if not put to meaningful use. Therefore, in this section electronic principles and component details will be applied to the operation of functional electronic units. Those units to be discussed are power supplies, detectors, amplifiers, and readout devices.

CHAPTER 11

POWER SUPPLIES

The variety of functions performed by instruments requires diverse power sources that produce an assortment of voltage levels of alternating and direct current. The power supply provides an instrument's circuit with various levels of ac voltage. This is accomplished by the transformer action previously discussed. Thus, available to the circuit are stepped-up and stepped-down voltages. The power supply also provides required direct current. Direct current is obtained through the rectification of alternating current in the power supply.

Most instruments contain within their design and construction an electronic power supply. Characteristically, electronic power supplies consist of five stages: transformer, rectifier, filter, voltage regulator, and voltage divider (Fig. 11-1).

TRANSFORMER

The transformer functions to step up and/or step down input ac voltage supplied from commercial power generators. This is accomplished through the induction of current in the primary winding of the transformer. Transformer construction and operational principles are detailed in Chapter 9.

RECTIFIER

The rectifier converts alternating current into unidirectional or direct current. Both half-wave and full-wave rectifiers produce pulsating direct current that requires additional processing to be transformed into uniformly constant direct current. Design and operation of the rectifying component, the diode, are discussed in Chapter 10.

FILTER

The filter network converts pulsating direct current to smooth direct current. The variation in dc pulsating voltage is called "ripple." When a direct current is required, ripple is undesirable and must be removed. Ripple is removed by

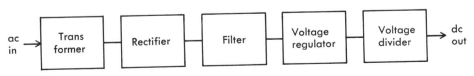

Fig. 11-1. Five stages of an electronic power supply.

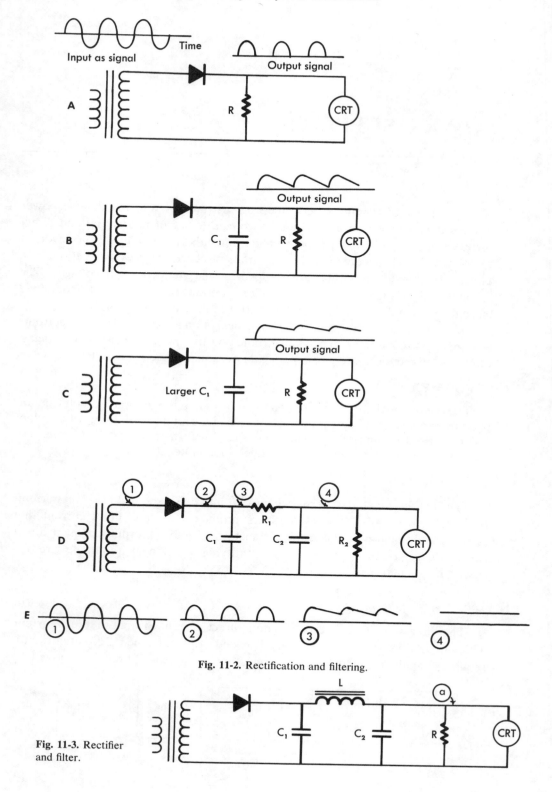

Fig. 11-2. Rectification and filtering.

Fig. 11-3. Rectifier and filter.

filtering. To convert pulsating dc to smooth, constant dc, a device is needed that will store current during the conduction part of the cycle and release it during the nonconduction part of the cycle of the diode. The capacitor is capable of storing and releasing a charge and is, therefore, an important component in the filtering process. A circuit containing a rectifier and a filtering network is shown in Fig. 11-2. Follow carefully the explanation of this circuit given below.

Refer to Fig. 11-2, *A*. Shown is a half-wave rectifier with no filtering. The output of the circuit is viewed by the CRT connected across R. As explained in the discussion of rectification, when the diode is forward biased, it conducts and a voltage is registered on the CRT. When the diode is reverse biased, it does not conduct and in effect opens the circuit, preventing current flow. Therefore, the CRT shows no output voltage when the input ac voltage is in the negative half of the waveform.

In Fig. 11-2, *B*, to the half-wave rectifier system is added a capacitor (C_1) in parallel to R. When the diode is conducting, the capacitor will be charged. When the conduction of the diode begins to decline, the capacitor will discharge through R. This discharging of the capacitor will in effect "fill in the voltage gap" left when the diode is not conducting.

Now refer to Fig. 11-2, *C*. The capacitor in *B* is replaced by a larger capacitor. The larger capacitor is capable of storing a larger charge; therefore, the discharge can fill in the voltage gap better than the discharge from the first capacitor.

Refer to Fig. 11-2, *D*. Two capacitors, C_1 and C_2, are used in the filtering system. In this case, capacitance has been increased by placing two capacitors in parallel. Also, an added feature for consideration is the capability of having two different RC charging and discharging time constants. C_1 charges, then discharges through R_1. C_2 "sees" a pulsating current of lesser variation than was "seen" by C_1. It is the task of C_2 to further smooth out the ripple by discharging at such a rate as to fill in the "small dip" still seen in the voltage.

In Fig. 11-2, *E*, the changes occuring in the input ac voltage as it passes through the circuit in *D* are designated as numbered points in the circuit. This, in effect, represents the metamorphosis of ac voltage to dc voltage.

In Fig. 11-3, an inductor has replaced R_1 Fig. 11-2, *D*. An inductor and a capacitor can be used in a power supply circuit to effect filtering. In this circuit, the current flow increasing through the inductor develops a voltage. The polarity of the voltage induced opposes the source voltage and tends to decrease the current. The magnetic field developed by the changing current flow (ripple portion of the current) in the inductor is actually stored energy that is extracted from the source. When the source voltage decreases, the magnetic field around the inductor collapses. The collapsing lines of force cut across the windings of the coil and induce current, which tends to maintain current flow in the original direction. In other words, the inductor stores energy when the diode is conducting (current increasing) and releases energy back into the circuit when the current decreases. As the magnetic field around the coils "pulsates," current is hindered or supplied to the circuit in such a way as to aid in smoothing the ripple in the dc pulsating current.

Several stages of filter networks can be used to obtain almost pure direct current, that is, direct current with extremely low values of ripple. Frequently, electrolytic capacitors are used because of their high capacitances.

For simplicity, in the foregoing examples a half-wave rectifier was used in the circuits. Capacitors and inductors must be large in these cases because of the need for stored energy over a long period of time. In other words, a large voltage gap must be filled. If a full-wave rectifier were substituted, several desirable goals would be achieved. First, both halves of the ac input sine wave would be used, thus almost doubling the efficiency of the power supply. Next, the diodes would be conducting more frequently, the total current provided by each would be less, and the diodes would last longer because of less wear. Finally, because the inductors and the capacitors would be used for filtering the power supply current for a shorter period of time, they would be smaller and less expensive.

In the above discussion about semiconductor power supplies, all points are equally applicable to vacuum tube power supplies.

VOLTAGE REGULATOR

Constant dc current output would be obtained from power supplies if the ac input were always constant. Unfortunately, line voltage fluctuations frequently occur. A fluctuation in the voltage input to the transformer results in a fluctuation in the power supply voltage output.

If instrument functional units require constant dc voltage with narrow tolerances, the voltage output from the power supply must be regulated. Voltage regulation is obtained with three types of voltage regulators: zener diode, gas-filled diode (glow tube), and electronic.

The purpose of voltage regulation is to maintain a constant voltage even during changes in current. Consider point a in Fig. 11-3. If voltage at this point must be maintained at a constant level, how can this be achieved if current increases in this circuit? Ohm's law provides three factors with which to work — current (I), voltage (E), and resistance (R). Therefore, if E must remain constant and I increases, then R must decrease as stipulated by the equation: $E = IR$. Thus, by replacing the resistor, R, with an electronic component with the capability of responding to current change in such a way that its effective resistance will be increased or decreased with current decrease or increase, respectively, voltage can be maintained at a constant level. This is essentially how each of the three voltage regulators operates to maintain a constant voltage at point a.

Fig. 11-4 shows the circuit in Fig. 11-3 with R replaced by a zener diode. The function of the zener diode was beiefly discussed in Chapter 10. Current will flow through a reverse-biased zener diode when the breakdown voltage (zener voltage) is applied across the diode. Zener diodes are designed and constructed to operate at any specific breakdown voltage required. Point a in Fig. 11-4 is maintained at a constant voltage through the operation of the zener diode. If the voltage increases to the level of the breakdown voltage of the zener diode, current flows through the zener diode, thus dropping the excess voltage across the zener diode while maintaining a constant voltage at point a.

Gas-filled diodes can be used to maintain a constant voltage. The effective

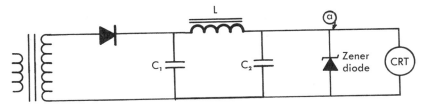

Fig. 11-4. Rectifier and filter with zener diode voltage regulator.

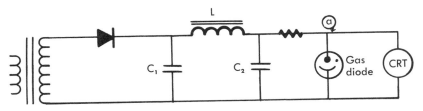

Fig. 11-5. Rectifier and filter with gas diode voltage regulator.

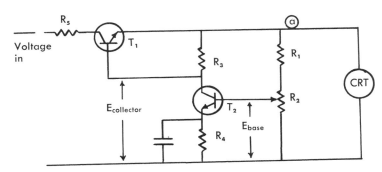

Fig. 11-6. Electronic voltage regulator.

resistance of a gas-filled diode is determined by ionization of the gas contained within the tube. (In the symbolic representation of a gas diode shown in Fig. 11-5, the dot indicates that the tube contains a gas.) The tube exerts infinite resistance when the gas is not ionized and an extremely low resistance when the gas is ionized. Ionization of the gas occurs after a certain potential (the triggering potential level depends upon the tube design) is applied across the tube. As a result of ionization, the tube conducts current, allowing a potential to be dropped across the tube. Thus, in Fig. 11-5, a constant voltage is maintained at point *a* through the responsiveness of the gas diode to an increase in voltage at point *a*.

An electronic voltage regulator will be briefly described, although an understanding of its operation may not be realized fully until after the discussion of triodes and transistors in Chapter 13. Fig. 11-6 shows an electronic voltage regulator containing two NPN transistors. An increase of voltage at point *a* results in an increased current through resistors R_1 and R_2 and, therefore, an increased voltage on the base of T_2. The more positive base causes T_2 to conduct more current (effective resistance decreased). As a result, the voltage on the base of T_1

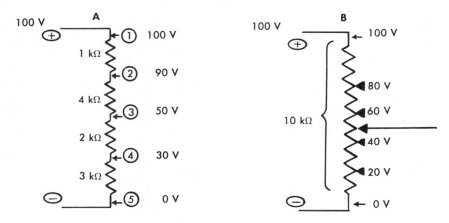

Fig. 11-7. Voltage divider.

is decreased, causing it to conduct less current (effective resistance increased). Through this type of feedback control system, a constant voltage is maintained at point *a*.

VOLTAGE DIVIDER

The application of voltage division enables a power supply to provide required dc voltages to different circuits within an instrument. As shown in Fig. 11-7, different voltages may be obtained by dropping voltage across a series of resistors. Voltage may also be varied by using a potentiometer. Voltage division and resistor components have been discussed in detail in Chapters 5 and 6.

INSTRUCTIONAL ACTIVITIES

1. Display a zener diode, a transistor, and a gas-filled diode.
2. Demonstrate rectification and filtering in a power supply. Build the circuit shown in Fig. 11-2, *D*, and, using an oscilloscope, show the waveforms at the four designated points.
3. Demonstrate voltage regulation.
   Using a variable dc voltage source, a resistor, a zener diode, and a VOM, build the circuit shown below:

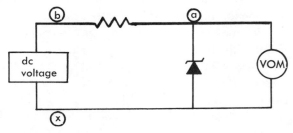

Demonstrate that voltage can be maintained at a constant level at point A even when the input dc voltage is increased. Changes in the dc voltage from the variable dc voltage source must be kept within the operational range of the particular zener diode being used. Measurement of the voltages at points *a* and *b* should be taken with reference to point *x*.

CHAPTER 12

DETECTORS

The quantification of biological fluid constituents in a sample being analyzed is based upon the detection of characteristic properties of the sample. The method of detection in clinical laboratory analytical instruments is primarily photo-detection, that is, detection of light or radiant energy. Other methods of detection of more limited application include temperature detection and gas composition detection. Although this list does not include all available detection methods, one of these three types of detectors is found in the majority of clinical laboratory instruments. Therefore, the discussion of detectors will be limited to these three types.

Each of the three types of detectors—photosensitive, temperature, and gas composition—differs in design, construction, and operational principle. However, the three types do have one characteristic in common: they are transducers. A transducer is a device that detects one form of energy and converts it to another form of energy. The detectors in clinical laboratory instruments usually detect a physical or chemical property—for example, light, heat, and gas molecules—and convert the physical or chemical energy into electrical energy. That electrical signal is then processed by a signal handling device. For example, the signal is usually amplified before being directed to a readout display.

PHOTOSENSITIVE DETECTORS

Photodetection is the basis of quantification in spectrophotometers, fluorom-eters, emission flame photometers, atomic absorption spectrophotometers, and optical cell counters. The photodetectors to be discussed include the barrier-layer cell, the phototube, the photomultiplier tube, and the semiconductor photo-diode. These photodetectors use photosensitive or photoemissive materials. A photosensitive material consists of atoms that release electrons when exposed to radiant energy. When light impinges upon the surface of a photosensitive material, electrons are freed by the radiant energy. The free electrons allow for electron flow (called photocurrent) when a closed circuit is provided. This principle is applicable to each of the photosensitive detectors to be discussed.

The barrier-layer cell (also called a photovoltaic cell) generates its electrical output directly from light energy. Therefore, it needs no external power source.

Construction of the barrier-layer cell is shown in Fig. 12-1. A thin layer of semiconductor, usually selenium, is deposited on a metal base, usually iron. The selenium is coated with a very thin transparent layer of silver lacquer. A glass protective window is placed over the lacquered surface, and the cell is encased in plastic. The iron acts as the positive electrode and the selenium as the negative electrode or collector. A wire lead extends through the plastic case from each of the two electrodes.

When light passes through the glass and the lacquer to impinge upon the selenium surface, enough energy is provided to the selenium to cause liberation of some electrons. The emitted electrons are collected by the silver lacquer. If the photovoltaic cell is connected in an unbroken circuit, electrons flow from the collector through the circuit to the iron electrode and finally back to the selenium. Thus, if an ammeter or a galvanometer is connected across the terminals of the photovoltaic cell, the current reading on the ammeter will be directly related to the intensity of radiant energy striking the cell's photosensitive surface.

The range of wavelengths of radiant energy to which a photodetector responds is referred to as its spectral response. The spectral response of a selenium photovoltaic cell with a protective glass window is about the same as the spectral response of the retina of the human eye. Radiant energy in the visible region (380 to 700 nm) is detected, with the greatest sensitivity being in the wavelength range of 500 to 600 nm (or the colors of green and yellow).

Radiant energy travels in a wave-form and is commonly described by its wavelength, which is the distance between the peaks of adjacent waves. This distance is given in nanometers (nm) or angstroms (Å). A nanometer is 10^{-9} meter, and an angstrom is 10^{-10} meter.

The selenium barrier-layer cell is used mainly in colorimeters or spectrophotometers when relatively high levels of illumination exist. Spectrophotometers with narrow bandpass requirements cannot use a barrier-layer photodetector because of the low level of radiant energy directed to the detector. The barrier-layer cell generates an electrical signal at a level sufficient for direct readout without prior amplification.

This photodetector is rugged, inexpensive, and useful for detection of relatively high levels of illumination. However, it is not suitable for use in more sophisticated instruments because it demonstrates the undesirable characteristics of being overly subject to fatigue, a high temperature coefficient, and a poor modulation ability. With continued exposure to radiant energy, the barrier-layer cell's output gradually falls from its initial output level. High levels of illumination accentuate this fatigue effect. A fatigued cell becomes less sensitive; therefore, it may not generate a photocurrent with ordinarily detectable low levels of illumination. This disadvantage can be minimized in a spectrophotometer by using a light shutter that permits light to strike the photocell only while readings are being taken with a cuvette inserted into the cuvette well. The selenium barrier-layer cell has a high temperature coefficient. Electrons are freed from the selenium by thermal energy. In other words, with a temperature rise the photodetector's output increases. To control this effect, once the instrument is turned

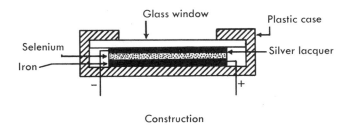

Construction

Schematic symbol

Fig. 12-1. Barrier-layer (photovoltaic) cell.

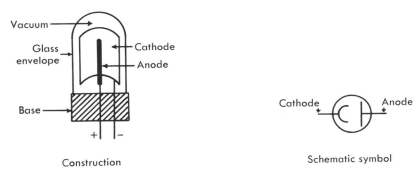

Construction

Schematic symbol

Fig. 12-2. Phototube.

on, readings should be taken only after the instrument has reached a constant temperature. The modulation ability of this photodetector is poor—that is, it responds sluggishly or not at all to changes in light intensity. The barrier-layer cell cannot respond to light interruptions of only 15 to 60 cycles per second.

Another photodetector is the phototube. A phototube consists of a curved sheet of photosensitive material that serves as an emitter or cathode and a positively charged thin tube that serves as a collector or anode. Both the cathode and anode are encased in an evacuated glass envelope. A dc potential applied to each electrode is provided by the instrument's power supply. Phototubes are commonly used in many photometric instruments. The phototube construction and schematic symbol are shown in Fig. 12-2.

The cathode of the phototube is coated with a photosensitive material that emits electrons when radiant energy impinges upon it. Cesium-antimony and multialkali (Sb/K/Na/Cs) are commonly used photosensitive materials. The spectral response depends upon the photosensitive material used on the cathode.

Because of its positive charge, the anode attracts or collects the electrons emitted from the cathode. A proportionality exists between the intensity of the radiant energy striking the cathode and the number of electrons emitted. In other words, the greater the intensity the more electrons emitted. The amount of photocurrent generated from the phototube is very small and must undergo considerable amplification before a usable signal is obtained.

The low level of photocurrent generated by this variety of phototube is at times a disadvantage. One approach to solving this problem is to increase the gain of the amplifier, thus increasing the current to the readout device. Another approach is to modify the phototube so that it will provide considerable amplification within itself. Two types of phototube modifications have been produced.

The first type is a gas-filled phototube. The tube is filled with a gas that is ionized by the electrons emitted from the cathode. Radiant energy striking the cathode liberates electrons that collide with, and cause ionization of, some gas atoms. The ionized gas atoms collide with and ionize other gas atoms, and the effect cascades. The overall effect of the ionization of gas atoms is to increase the total number of charged particles generated by radiant energy striking the cathode—that is, to amplify the generated signal. Gas-filled phototubes have poorer modulation ability, poorer stability, and shorter lives than vacuum phototubes.

The second approach to obtaining amplification within a phototube is to increase the number of electron-emitting electrodes within the tube. This modification resulted in the development of a photosensitive detector called a photomultiplier tube.

Figs. 12-3 and 12-4 show construction of, and schematic symbols for, the linear and circular design of photomultiplier tubes, respectively. The photomultiplier tube consists of a cathode, an anode, and nine to sixteen photosensitive electrodes, called dynodes, encased in an evacuated glass envelope. When radiant energy strikes the cathode, emitted electrons are focused on and attracted to the first dynode. On striking the dynode, the electrons cause the emission of a greater number of electrons than the number striking it. One primary electron can yield from three to six secondary electrons. The electrons emitted from dynode 1 are then focused and attracted to dynode 2, where the process is repeated. The chain reaction continues through the entire series of dynodes until the anode is reached. Because each dynode emits more electrons than strike it, an internal amplification results.

Electrons are focused and attracted from dynode to dynode in two ways. First, the dynodes are physically placed and shaped so that electrons tend to "bounce" toward the following dynode. Second, each successive dynode is maintained at a higher positive potential than its predecessor. Successive dynodes are operated at voltages increasing in equal steps of 30 to 100 V.

The internal amplification achieved by a photomultiplier tube can be as high as 10^6. In other words, the anode current may be as high as 10^6 times the original current generated at the cathode. By increasing the number of dynodes, it would seem that even greater amplification could be achieved. However, each succes-

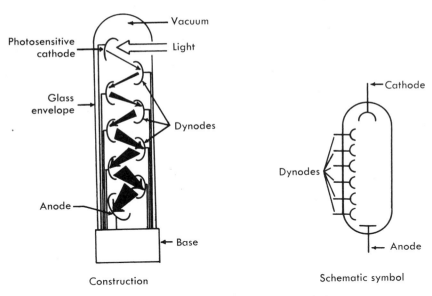

Fig. 12-3. Photomultiplier tube — linear type design.

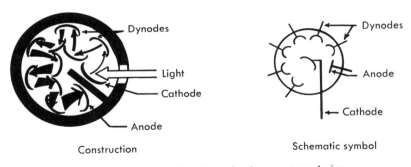

Fig. 12-4. Photomultiplier tube — circular cage type design.

sive dynode is at a higher positive potential. Therefore, with too many dynodes, voltage levels are impractical to achieve or are so high that arcing to dynodes of lower potential will occur. Normally, the number of dynodes in a photomultiplier tube is limited to a maximum of 16.

The required dynode voltages are usually obtained from a resistor-voltage divider network across which is applied a high positive voltage from the power supply (Fig. 12-5).

The sensitivity and the response time of the photomultiplier tube are far superior to those of the phototube. Light intensities 200 times weaker than those that can be detected by a phototube and amplifier can be measured by a photomultiplier tube. The photomultiplier tube can respond to light interruptions of 10^9 per second.

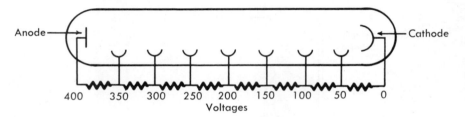

Fig. 12-5. Voltage divider network supplying dynode voltages for photomultiplier tube.

The photoemissive surfaces in the photomultiplier tube have three general characteristics worthy of review. First, the number of emitted electrons per unit of time is directly proportional to the light intensity impinging upon the photoemissive surface. Second, the energy of the released electrons, independent of the intensity of light, depends upon the frequency of the radiant energy. Therefore, a tube may respond differently at different wavelengths. A tube that responds well to visible light wavelengths may not respond satisfactorily to shorter or longer wavelengths. Photomultiplier tubes made with different photoemissive materials are selectively responsive to specific wavelength ranges of radiant energy. Third, the delayed response in a photomultiplier tube is caused by delays encountered in the associated circuitry outside the tube. Electron emission resulting from radiant energy absorption is virtually instantaneous.

Photomultiplier tubes should not be exposed to extraneous light while voltage is being applied to them. For example, their protective covers should not be removed. If exposed to intense light, the cathode will emit more electrons than it can replace, and the tube will fatigue. The cathode may recover from the fatigue effect if stored in the dark for a period of time. However, strong intensity and prolonged exposure may destroy the integrity of the cathode.

Instruments containing phototubes or photomultiplier tubes should not be operated in an environment characterized by low temperature and high humidity. In this type of environment, condensation is likely to occur on the tube's surface. Condensation on the glass envelope will diminish the amount of light allowed to impinge upon the photoemissive cathode, resulting in erroneous output signals.

The fourth photodetector to be described briefly is the semiconductor photodiode. This photodetector is a specifically processed silicon P-N junction that converts radiant energy into electron flow. When radiant energy impinges upon the P-N junction, valence electrons acquire energy that enables them to move. Movement of electrons constitutes current flow. Thus, the intensity of radiant energy striking the photodiode is directly related to the output current. Characteristics of the photodiode are such that the current generated is reverse current. Therefore, a photodiode must be reverse biased to function as a photodetector.

TEMPERATURE DETECTOR

Osmolality is a clinically useful determination of the number of particles in biological fluids. An instrument called an osmometer is used to determine osmolal-

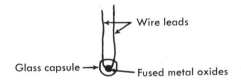

Fig. 12-6. Thermistor.

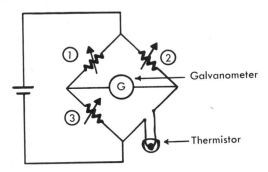

Fig. 12-7. Thermistor in Wheatstone bridge circuit.

ities. Measuring the freezing point depression of specimens being analyzed is one method used in osmolality determination. A solution's freezing point decreases as the number of particles suspended in it increases. Therefore, temperature detection is used in this instrument to quantify the number of particles in a solution. The detector is called a thermistor.

A thermistor is a temperature measuring device consisting of a small button, constructed of a fused mixture of metal oxides, that is attached to two leads and encapsulated in glass (Fig. 12-6). The metal oxide mixture (for example, manganese, nickel, copper, and uranium) possesses a very large negative temperature coefficient of resistance. A small decrease in temperature causes a relatively large increase in the resistance of the thermistor. For example, at 50°C a thermistor may have one fifth the resistance it had at 25°C. This large change in resistance and the thermistor's small size make this device a useful temperature detector with particular applications for small amounts of material.

A temperature change results in a proportional change in the resistance of the thermistor. Therefore, temperature can be measured by measuring the thermistor's resistance. This resistance is measured by a Wheatstone bridge circuit (Fig. 12-7). With the thermistor at a standard temperature, the three variable resistors are adjusted to balance the circuit—that is, no current is flowing through the galvanometer. Once the circuit is balanced, the thermistor can be used to measure a temperature change. As the temperature changes, the thermistor's resistance will change and a current will flow through the galvanometer. The current then can be related to resistance change and, therefore, to temperature change.

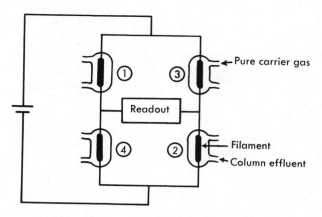

Fig. 12-8. Thermal conductivity detector.

GAS DETECTORS

A gas chromatograph is an instrument used in the clinical laboratory to separate, isolate, identify, and quantify chemically related compounds in a vaporized solution. The solution to be analyzed is vaporized and carried through a column by the constant flow of an inert gas. The column is of specific design and composition and functions to delay selectively the different compounds in the sample vapor. Therefore, the compounds pass into the detector at times characteristic of their chemical and/or physical properties. Identification of the compound is based upon the time required for it to reach the detector. The detector's function is only to quantify the gas molecules passing through the detector. The detectors must be very sensitive because small samples are usually used. Detection of the separated gas molecules is accomplished by using one of three general methods—thermal conductivity, flame ionization, and electron capture.

Analysis by thermal conductivity is based upon the differences in thermal conductivity between a pure carrier gas and a gas containing larger and more numerous molecules. Thermal conductivity is the rate at which heat is carried through a gas. The thermal conductivity of the inert carrier gas is greater than that of the gas under analysis (effluent from the column) because the carrier gas contains faster molecules. If each of these gases were to flow at a constant rate over a heated filament, the carrier gas would cool the filament faster than the other gas would. The resistance of most metals increases with an increase in temperature. Therefore, the difference in the rates at which gases cool a metal filament can be measured as a resistance difference. This resistance difference can in turn be related to the molecular concentration of a particular vaporized sample.

Fig. 12-8 shows a thermal conductivity detector. A Wheatstone bridge circuit consists of four filaments with closely matched resistances. The pure carrier gas and the sample (effluent) from the column flow at a constant rate over filaments 3 and 4 and filaments 1 and 2, respectively. The bridge arrangement is enclosed in a temperature-regulated chamber. The filaments are heated by a constant cur-

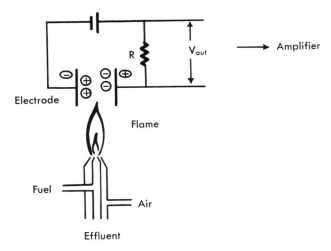

Fig. 12-9. Flame ionization detector.

rent. When a gas containing more molecules than are found in the carrier gas passes over filaments 1 and 2, the temperature, and therefore the resistance, of these filaments increases proportionately with the number of molecules in the gas. The Wheatsone bridge will be unbalanced, and a current will be amplified and then directed to the readout device. The amount of current is directly related to the relative molecular concentration of the sample.

The flame ionization detector is represented in Fig. 12-9. The operation of this highly sensitive detector is based upon the phenomenon that the combustion of organic compounds produces ionic fragmentation and free electrons. Ions and electrons between two oppositely charged electrodes will conduct a current between those electrodes.

The flame ionization detector consists of a hydrogen flame positioned between two electrodes across which is placed a high voltage. The column effluent is directed into the flame after being mixed with the hydrogen fuel. The support gas used for this flame is air. The ionic fragments and free electrons produced by the thermal energy of the flame serve as conductors of current between the two electrodes. The ions and electrons act to decrease the effective resistance between the electrodes. Therefore, with increased ions and electrons, there is decreased resistance and thus increased current through the circuit.

Current increase causes an increase in the voltage drop across R in Fig. 12-9. The output voltage is amplified before being directed to a readout device. The readout represents the amount of organic compound in the column effluent as reflected through current and voltage levels in the circuit of the flame ionization detector.

The electron-capture detector is the third type of detector used to quantify organic molecules in the column effluent. The operation of this detector is based upon the ability of large organic molecules, particularly halogens, to readily capture electrons to form negatively charged ions.

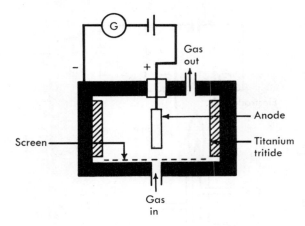

Fig. 12-10. Electron capture detector.

The construction of the electron-capture detector is represented in Fig. 12-10. The column effluent enters the detector by passing through a screen that smooths the gas flow through the chamber. Within the chamber are a cathode, an anode, and a source of beta particles (β^-), which are high-speed electrons emitted from the nucleus of an atom. The source of beta particles is a radioactive material such as titanium tritide. As the carrier gas of nitrogen or argon flows through the detector, the beta particles cause ionization of the gas molecules, producing electrons and positive ions. The electrons are attracted to the anode, while the large positive ions are usually swept out of the chamber before reaching the cathode and therefore contribute minimally to the current in the circuit. Measurement of the current is represented by the galvanometer designated G in Fig. 12-10. In actual practice, however, the current is amplified before being displayed on a readout device. During the flow of the carrier gas through the chamber, a constant current flows in the circuit.

When a column effluent containing organic molecules enters the chamber, the free electrons are captured by the organic molecules to form large negative ions. These large ions are slow moving and are usually swept from the chamber before reaching the anode. This results in fewer negative charges reaching the anode and, therefore, a decrease in the current in the circuit. The greater the number of organic molecules carried by the carrier gas in the effluent, the greater the number of electrons captured. With a decreased number of electrons attracted to the anode, there is a decreased current in the circuit. This method of gas molecule detection relates current indirectly to the quantity of organic molecules in the column effluent.

INSTRUCTIONAL ACTIVITIES

1. Display different types of detectors, for example, barrier-layer cell, phototube, photomultiplier tube, thermistor, thermal conductivity, flame ionization, and electron capture.
2. Have the students identify detectors found in commonly used clinical laboratory instruments.
3. Demonstrate the negative temperature coefficient of resistance of a thermistor. Mea-

sure the resistance across a thermistor at 0°C (ice bath), at room temperature, and at an increased temperature, for example, 30°C to 35°C. As the temperature is increased the resistance will decrease.

4. Demonstrate photocurrent production by radiant energy impinging upon the photosensitive surface of a barrier-layer cell. Connect a VOM across a barrier-layer cell. Note the voltage output of the cell when the photosensitive surface is exposed to different intensities of radiant energy.
The photocurrent will increase with increased intensity of radiant energy.

5. Demonstrate the effect of fatigue on the barrier-layer cell. Connect a VOM across a barrier-layer cell. Expose the photosensitive surface of the cell to a relatively intense light source. With prolonged exposure, the voltage generated by the cell will decrease.

6. Demonstrate the high temperature coefficuent of the barrier-layer cell. Connect a VOM across a barrier-layer cell with its photosensitive surface protected from radiant energy. Note the production of a current as the barrier-layer cell is heated.

7. Demonstrate the poor modulation ability of the barrier-layer cell. Connect a VOM across a barrier-layer cell, and direct a light at the photosensitive surface. Interrupt the light beam at specified frequencies, for example, 5 Hz, 10 Hz, 15 Hz, 30 Hz, and 60 Hz. Note the frequencies of those interruptions at which the barrier-layer cell does not respond maximally.

CHAPTER 13

AMPLIFIERS

A frequent requirement within instruments' electronic circuitry is amplification of a signal. In this chapter amplification will be defined, and various types of amplifiers will be described and their functions discussed.

AMPLIFICATION

As mentioned in previous chapters, output signals from detectors may be amplified before being directed to readout devices. Amplification is simply changing a small signal into a signal of larger amplitude — that is, magnifying it. A basic description of amplification is a small input signal affecting a circuit in such a way that a large output signal results.

Fig. 13-1 illustrates the concept of amplification. In the diagram, the voltage source (V_s) is a constant dc source, R_1 is a fixed resistor, and R_2 is a variable resistor. If the wiper arm of R_2 is moved upward, the R_2 resistance is decreased and, as a result, the output voltage (V_{out}) decreases. On the other hand, if the wiper arm on R_2 is moved downward, the resistance of R_2 increases and the out-

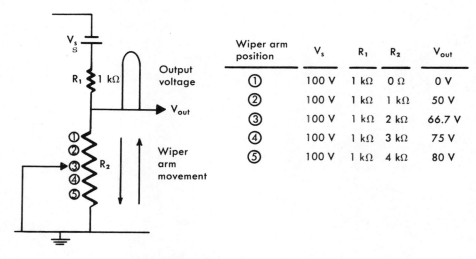

Wiper arm position	V_s	R_1	R_2	V_{out}
①	100 V	1 kΩ	0 Ω	0 V
②	100 V	1 kΩ	1 kΩ	50 V
③	100 V	1 kΩ	2 kΩ	66.7 V
④	100 V	1 kΩ	3 kΩ	75 V
⑤	100 V	1 kΩ	4 kΩ	80 V

Fig. 13-1. Conceptual amplification.

put voltage increases. This concept of amplification is an application of voltage division discussed earlier in Chapters 2 and 5.

Consider a hypothetical situation. In Fig. 13-1 the fixed resistor value is 1 kΩ, the variable resistor can be adjusted from 0 Ω to 4 kΩ in increments of 1 kΩ, and the voltage source is 100 V. Calculate the output voltage for each of the five indicated positions of the wiper arm. As is clearly shown with this example, a change in the resistance of R_2 results in a change in voltage output.

If R_2 is very sensitive, a small change in the wiper arm position produces a large change in resistance. Therefore, a small movement of the R_2 wiper arm would result in a large voltage change at the output. This is essentially how a small input voltage affects a vacuum tube or semiconductor transistor amplifier. With the change of the input voltage amplitude, there is a large change in the effective resistance of the amplifier, resulting in a large change in the output voltage. Exactly how an input voltage change is expressed as a change in effective resistance will be clarified in the discussion of operational principles of amplifiers, which follows later in this chapter.

The degree of amplification of a signal by an amplifier is referred to as the *gain* of the amplifier. Gain is the ratio of output voltage to input voltage:

$$Gain = V_{out}/V_{in}$$

If an input voltage of 0.1 V results in an output voltage of 10 V, the gain of the amplifier is 100, as calculated below:

$$Gain = V_{out}/V_{in} = 10 \text{ V}/0.1 \text{ V} = 100$$

Several types of amplifiers have been developed, including vacuum tube, semiconductor, and operational amplifiers. Construction, schematic representation, and operational principles of each type will be briefly discussed.

VACUUM TUBES

Vacuum tube operational principles were included in the discussion of the vacuum tube diode in Chapter 10. Since these operational principles are the basis upon which vacuum tube amplifiers function, review of this previous material may be beneficial. Both rectification and amplification may be achieved through the application of these basic vacuum tube principles. Rectification results from the action of a diode. Amplification can be obtained by using vacuum tubes, including triodes, tetrodes, and pentodes.

A triode consists of the same components as a diode with the addition of one element called a control grid. Thus, a triode consists of a cathode, a plate, a heater, and a control grid, all of which are encased within an evacuated glass envelope. The control grid is a wire helically wound around the cathode. The grid is positioned between the cathode and plate, closer to the cathode than to the plate. Fig. 13-2 shows the schematic symbol used for a triode vacuum tube. The presence of a heater is assumed when not specifically indicated in schematic representations of vacuum tubes.

Fig. 13-3 illustrates the operation of a vacuum tube triode. As in a forward-

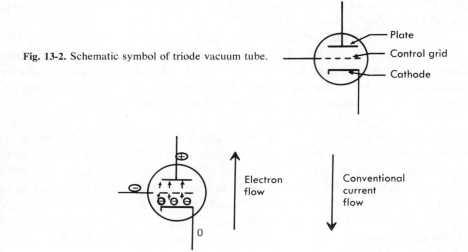

Fig. 13-2. Schematic symbol of triode vacuum tube.

Plate

Control grid

Cathode

Electron flow

Conventional current flow

Fig. 13-3. Operation of triode vacuum tube.

biased vacuum tube diode, electrons are emitted from the heated cathode and are attracted to the positively charged plate. Conventional current flows through the tube from the plate to the cathode. Current through the tube is called plate current.

Electron flow from the cathode to the plate is controlled by the control grid. When the control grid of the triode is made increasingly more negative with respect to the cathode, repulsion of the electrons by the grid results in fewer electrons reaching the positively charged plate. Thus, with an increase of the negative grid potential, there is an increase in the effective resistance (effective resistance of a vacuum tube is called plate resistance) of the tube and a decrease in the plate current.

An operationally biased triode is one in which the plate is considerably more positive and the control grid slightly more negative than the cathode. A small ac signal applied to the control grid continuously alters the grid bias, thus changing the current through the tube and consequently the voltage on the plate. The voltage output taken at the plate will have a waveform 180° out of phase with, and of greater amplitude than, the waveform of the input signal on the control grid. This production of a large output signal by a small input signal is called amplification.

Fig. 13-4 represents a triode vacuum tube amplifier that is functionally comparable to the circuit shown in Fig. 13-1. As the small input signal applied to the negatively-biased control grid swings in the positive direction, the grid becomes less negative, the plate resistance decreases, the plate current increases, and the output voltage decreases. When the input signal swings in the negative direction, the grid becomes more negative, the plate resistance increases, the plate current decreases, and the output voltage increases.

In summary, the small input voltage continuously alters the control grid bias

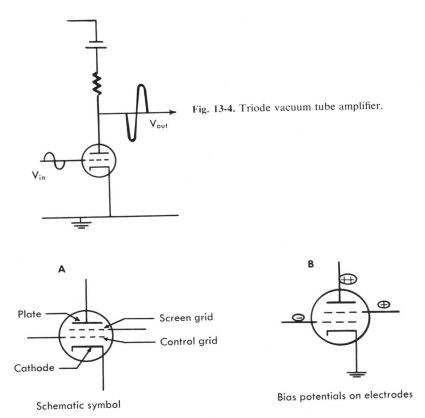

Fig. 13-4. Triode vacuum tube amplifier.

V_{out}

V_{in}

A

Plate

Cathode

Screen grid

Control grid

Schematic symbol

B

Bias potentials on electrodes

Fig. 13-5. Tetrode vacuum tube.

in respect to the cathode, which changes the conductivity or resistance of the tube, which affects the plate current, which determines the output voltage. The process of amplification is a dynamic expression of Ohm's law.

Two other vacuum tubes used for amplification are the tetrode and the pentode. The operational principle of each is essentially the same as that of the triode. First, the triode was modified to form a tetrode; later, a modification of the tetrode produced the pentode.

The tetrode is a four-element vacuum tube developed by adding a screen grid to the triode. The screen grid is located between the control grid and the plate (Fig. 13-5, *A*) and is maintained at a positive dc potential (Fig. 13-5, *B*). In the triode, unwanted capacitance develops between the control grid and the plate. This capacitance is called interelectrode capacitance. The screen grid has two effects: (1) it reduces the grid-to-plate interelectrode capacitance and (2) since the screen grid is at a positive potential, it attracts the electrons emitted from the cathode, serving to accelerate them toward the plate.

The impact of the highly accelerated electrons upon the plate results in the emission of electrons from the plate. The cathode emission of electrons is called

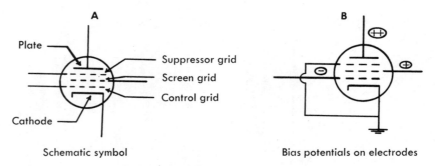

Fig. 13-6. Pentode vacuum tube.

primary emission; therefore, the emission of electrons from the plate is called secondary emission. Electrons freed as a result of secondary emission are attracted to the electrode of highest positive potential. When the plate voltage is high, the electrons contribute to the plate current. However, when the plate voltage is at its minimum value, the electrons are attracted to the screen grid, resulting in a screen grid current. This latter occurrence is undesirable, since amplification of the output signal is diminished with the decrease in possible plate current. This problem was solved by modifying the tetrode and thus developing the pentode.

The pentode vacuum tube contains a suppressor grid between the screen grid and the plate (Fig. 13-6, *A*). The suppressor grid is connected to the cathode, providing it with a potential that repels the secondary emission electrons back to the plate. Fig. 13-6, *B,* shows the bias potentials on an operational pentode. In effect, the suppressor grid eliminates excess screen grid current and enhances amplification.

SEMICONDUCTOR TRANSISTORS

Vacuum tubes have been virtually eliminated with the development and use of solid-state electronic devices. Two of these, the semiconductor diode and the semiconductor transistor, have replaced the vacuum tube diode and the amplifier, respectively. This innovation brought with it a number of advantages. Transistors are much smaller than vacuum tubes and have contributed to miniaturization in electronics. Warm-up time is eliminated in solid state electronics because, unlike vacuum tubes, transistors do not require heating filaments. Lower operating voltages are needed by transistors; therefore, smaller power supplies can be used. Transistors are less susceptible to breakage than vacuum tubes. Solid-state circuits are less expensive and last longer than equivalent vacuum tube circuits.

Vacuum tubes and transistors both function in amplification; however, their principles of operation differ. The crystalline structure and conducting characteristics of semiconductor materials were discussed in Chapter 10. The P-N junction semiconductor is the simplest of semiconductor functional electronic devices. Construction, operation, and application of the semiconductor diode were de-

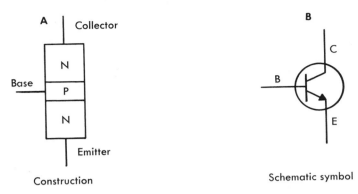

Fig. 13-7. NPN transistor.

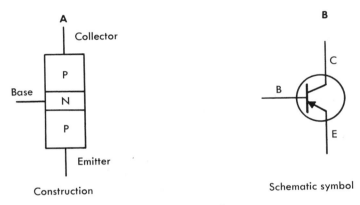

Fig. 13-8. PNP transistor.

scribed in Chapter 10 and should be reviewed prior to the presentation of semi-conductor transistors.

The origin of the name "transistor" represents the operation and the functional application of the device. When this semiconductor device was first developed in 1948, it was recognized that its resistance could be changed to regulate current flow in a circuit. The device was initially called a "transfer resistor," a functional description that soon became "transistor."

The first semiconductor transistors to be developed were junction transistors of two types, NPN and PNP. These transistors are called "junction transistors" because charge movement through them is regulated at the junction between fused negative or positive semiconductor materials. An NPN transistor consists of two N-type semiconductor wafers between which is fused a P-type semi-conductor (Fig. 13-7, *A*). N-type semiconductor material sandwiched between two P-type semiconductor wafers makes a PNP transistor (Fig. 13-8, *A*). The middle semiconductor material layer is very thin (approximately 0.001 inch thick) in each type of transistor and is called the base (B). The other two semiconductor elements in the transistor are called the collector (C) and the emitter (E). Schematic symbols for NPN and PNP transistors are shown in Figs. 13-7, *B*, and 13-8, *B*, respectively.

The base of the transistor is functionally equivalent to the control grid of the vacuum tube. The emitter is equivalent to the cathode, and the collector is equivalent to the plate. The base potential regulates the current flow through the transistor as the control grid potential regulates the current through the vacuum tube triode, tetrode, or pentode.

The direction of conventional current flow through a transistor is indicated by the emitter arrows in the schematic symbol. Current flow through the transistor is regulated by the base-to-emitter bias potential. The base exerts its control on electron flow in the NPN transistor and on "hole" or positive charge flow in the PNP transistor. The emitter is the source of free electrons and "holes" in NPN and PNP transistors, respectively. The collector is the electrode that attracts electrons and holes in NPN and PNP transistors, respectively.

To avoid confusion, it must be emphasized that charge flow through a transistor is from emitter to collector. In the NPN transistor, electrons flow from the emitter into the base region and then to the collector. In the PNP transistor, holes, or conceptually positive charges, flow from the emitter into the base material and then to the cathode. Movement of charges in the direction indicated above is achieved by biasing the electrodes of the transistors—that is, applying fixed dc potentials of different levels on each of the three electrodes. Transistors must be correctly biased to allow current flow. If a positive potential is applied to the P-type semiconductor and a negative potential is applied to the N-type semiconductor, the P-N junction will be forward biased. The P-N junction will be reverse biased if a positive potential is applied to the N-type semiconductor and a negative potential is applied to the P-type semiconductor. The standard operational fixed bias applied to junction semiconductor transistor amplifiers will cause the emitter-base junction to be forward biased and the base-collector junction to be reverse biased, as shown in Fig. 13-9.

Refer to Fig. 13-9, *A*, and follow the explanation of current flow through a properly biased NPN transistor. The negative potential at the emitter repels electrons toward the positively charged base. The majority of the electrons pass

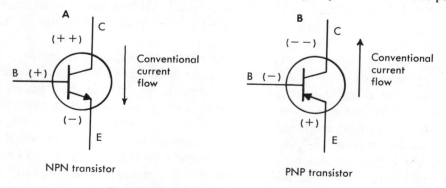

Fig. 13-9. Biasing of PNP and NPN transistors.

through the very thin base region to the collector, which is at a high positive potential. Current flow through a PNP transistor differs only slightly from that through an NPN transistor (Fig. 13-9, *B*). In the PNP transistor, the charges moved through the transistor are holes (positive charges) instead of electrons, as is the case in NPN transistors. The positive potential on the emitter of the PNP transistor repels the holes into the base region. The majority of these holes are attracted by the high negative potential on the collector and pass through the thin base region to the collector. Regulation of current flow is accomplished by regulating the emitter-base bias in both NPN and PNP transistors. Therefore, if the emitter potential remains unchanged, the potential on the base will regulate current flow through the transistor. This characteristic allows for the application of transistors to amplification.

The principle of amplification was considered in the presentation of vacuum tubes. Since the principle of amplification by transistors is similar to the principle of amplification by vacuum tubes, it will be mentioned only briefly here. In an NPN transistor, with a change in the emitter-base bias, current flow through the transistor is changed, and with a change in current flow through the transistor, the voltage at point *a* in Fig. 13-10 (that is, output voltage) is changed. An input signal is introduced at the base. As the base becomes more positive with respect to the emitter, more electrons are attracted by the base and more current flows in the circuit. With increased current, there is a greater voltage drop over R, and the voltage at point *a* decreases. When the input signal swings negative, the emitter-base bias is decreased, decreasing current flow, and therefore less voltage is dropped across R. In this case, the voltage at point *a* increases.

Refer to Fig. 13-11, and follow the explanation of amplification using a PNP transistor. An input signal is applied to the base. As the base becomes more positive with respect to the emitter, fewer holes are attracted to the base (essentially, the transistor's effective resistance is increased) and the voltage drop across the transistor is increased, resulting in a decreased voltage at point *a*. As

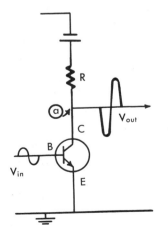
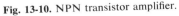

Fig. 13-10. NPN transistor amplifier.

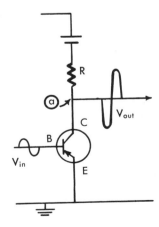

Fig. 13-11. PNP transistor amplifier.

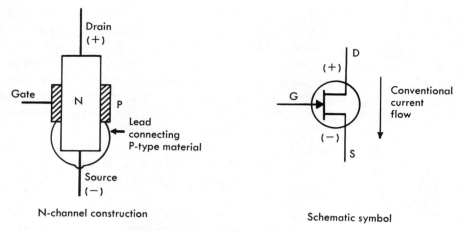

N-channel construction   Schematic symbol

Fig. 13-12. Field effect transistor (FET).

the input signal swings negative, holes are strongly attracted to the base region and then to the collector. This results in decreased effective resistance of the transistor, increased current flow through the transistor, decreased voltage drop across the transistor, and increased voltage at point *a*. Note that, as is the case with the vacuum tube amplifiers, a small input signal produces an output signal of greater amplitude that is 180° out of phase with the input signal.

The junction transistors discussed above are of limited usefulness when a signal must be amplified with minute current drain from the signal source. For example, a barrier-layer cell produces a photocurrent as a result of radiant energy striking a photosensitive material. To amplify the output signal from the barrier-layer cell, the amplifier must be able to produce a greater output signal without drawing much current from the barrier-layer cell. If substantial current were drawn from the barrier-layer cell, the cell would become fatigued, since the electrons would not be returned to the photosensitive material at a sufficient rate. Therefore, for limited current drain from voltage sources, an amplifier with a high input impedance must be used.

A semiconductor amplifier developed to provide a high input impedance is the field effect transistor (FET). Frequently, an FET is used as the first stage (that is, at the input) of a multistage amplifier. (A multistage amplifier consists of many individual amplifying transistors connected collector-to-base in series, with each transistor amplifying the output signal of the previous one.)

Field effect transistors are of two types, N-channel and P-channel. The construction and the schematic symbol of an N-channel semiconductor FET are shown in Fig. 13-12. The FET consists of a bar of semiconductor material called the channel, which is N-type or P-type depending upon whether the FET is N-channel or P-channel. An electrode is connected to each end of the channel. These electrodes are called the source (S) and the drain (D). The N-channel is fused between two layers of P-type semiconductor that are electrically connected.

To the P-type semiconductor is attached an electrode called the gate (G). Some FETs are designed with a gate consisting of a sleeve of P-type material around the N-channel.

FET operation closely parallels the operation of a vacuum tube triode. The effective resistance of the FET is controlled by the potential applied to the gate. In the N-channel, the electrons flow from the negatively charged source to the positively charged drain. When a negative voltage is applied to the gate, electron flow through the N-channel is hindered. The greater the negative potential on the gate, the greater the impedance to electron flow. Thus current flow decreases.

The advantage of very high input impedance has been enhanced with the development of the insulated-gate FET, or the metal oxide semiconductor field effect transistor (MOSFET). This modified FET consists of a gate insulated from the channel by a film of insulating metal oxide. As in the FET, the gate's electrostatic field controls charge flow through the channel. The MOSFET exerts the highest input impedance (as high as 10^{10} Ω) of any transistor.

The evolution of electronic devices, which has led to the development of the vacuum tube and the specifically designed semiconductor, continues. Discrete transistors and associated circuitry are being replaced by integrated circuits. An integrated circuit (IC) is a functional electronic circuit incorporated into a tiny piece of silicon, referred to as a "chip." Diodes, transistors, FETs, resistors, capacitors, and associated connections can be built into very small silicon chips. With the development of integrated circuits, miniaturization in electronics is frequently limited only by the requirement that connecting leads extend to the exterior of the protective cover of the IC.

The availability of ICs for a wide variety of applications has rapidly increased while the cost has decreased. Repair of ICs is difficult if not impossible; therefore, they are usually replaced rather than repaired. Such disposable electronic circuits are feasible because they are relatively inexpensive. Integrated circuits are being used increasingly in clinical laboratory instruments. A recent development in integrated circuits is the large-scale integrated circuit (LSI), which is an IC chip containing an entire instrument circuit or a large portion of it. LSI circuitry permits microminiaturization of instruments. Digital computers and small calculators are the first instruments to contain the LSI circuit.

OPERATIONAL AMPLIFIERS

The operational amplifier (OA or op amp) is a multistage amplifier system contained within one small unit or package. Like the solid-state devices discussed earlier, the op amp is replaced rather than repaired. The name "operational amplifier" was derived from its intended function of performing mathematical "operations" on a signal or signals. The flexibility and versatility of the op amp provide for a multitude of applications, some of which are utilized in the signal processing units of clinical laboratory instruments. A few of the many mathematical operations performed by the op amp include addition, subtraction, integration, differentiation, logarithm derivation, antilogarithm derivation, multiplication, and division.

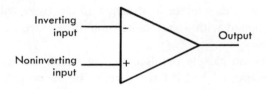

Fig. 13-13. Operational amplifier schematic symbol.

The op amp unit is available in different shapes and sizes, each having several (eight to sixteen) terminals. These terminals are connected to biasing voltages and associated circuitry. The terminals to be referred to in this brief discussion are the two input terminals and the one output terminal. As shown in Fig. 13-13, the output terminals are conventionally marked − and + for inverting input and noninverting input, respectively. A signal applied to the inverting input produces a signal of the opposite sign at the output − that is, the input signal is inverted. If a signal is applied to the noninverting input, the output signals have the same sign.

The function performed by an op amp is determined by the external associated circuitry. Fig. 13-14 shows a commonly used amplifier circuit that amplifies the input signal. The op amp has a large input impedance of at least 10^5 Ω and a high gain of at least 10^4. The gain of an operational amplifier circuit is calculated as follows:

$$\text{Gain}_{\text{op amp}} = R_2/R_1$$

where:

R_1 = Resistance of input resistor
R_2 = Feedback resistance

Examples of mathematical operations performed by op amp circuits will be presented with reference to Fig. 13-15. A detailed understanding of the operation of each sample op amp circuit is not expected. The examples are provided only to demonstrate the versatility of the op amp in performing different functions by changing and/or rearranging associated circuit components.

Addition of signals is achieved by establishing a circuit with a resistor in the feedback loop at *b* and parallel resistors at *a*, with each resistor conducting one of the input signals to be added. The output of the op amp will be the negative sum of the input signals.

Two signals can be subtracted in an op amp circuit by placing a resistor at *b* and two parallel resistors at *a*, with one input signal having a positive sign and the other a negative sign.

Integration is achieved in an op amp circuit that has a resistor at *a* and a capacitor at *b*. Measurement of area is obtained through the operation of integration.

Differentiation is obtained by exchanging the components in the integration circuit. Thus, a differentiator op amp circuit has a capacitor at *a* and a resistor at *b*. Measurement of slope or rate change is achieved through the operation of differentiation.

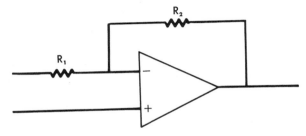

Fig. 13-14. Common operational amplifier circuit.

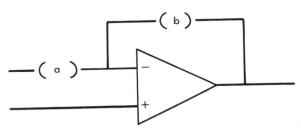

Fig. 13-15. Operational amplifier; optional associated circuitry for mathematical operations.

A logarithmic function is obtained from a log op amp circuit, which has a resistor at *a* and a P-N junction diode in a forward-biased orientation at *b*. This operation makes possible the direct conversion of transmittance to absorbance in spectrophotometry.

Antilogarithms can be obtained from an op amp circuit with a forward-biased P-N junction diode at *a* and a resistor at *b*.

Multiplication and division are more complex operations and require the application of three op amp circuits. To multiply or divide, first the logarithms of the variables are obtained. Then these logs are added for multiplication or subtracted for division, and finally, the antilogarithms are extracted.

The modular design of modern instrumentation has developed through the use of operational amplifiers and integrated circuitry. Since operational amplifiers have a multiplicity of applications, they are found in most instruments in which signal handling, simple or complex, is required. In clinical laboratory instruments, the signal generated, or affected by, the sample being analyzed is processed through any number of signal manipulations before being presented to the read-out device.

INSTRUCTIONAL ACTIVITIES

1. Display different vacuum tubes, for example, triode, tetrode, and pentode. Expose the vacuum tube elements, and request that the students identify each element and describe its function in amplification.
2. Display an assortment of semiconductor devices, for example, junction transistors, FET, MOSFET, IC, and op amp.
3. Build the circuit shown below, and demonstrate the principle of amplification.

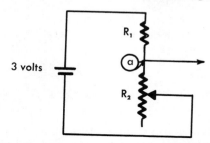

Using a VOM, demonstrate that the voltage at point *a* can be changed by adjusting the variable resistor R_2.

4. Build the circuit shown in Fig. 13-10. Using a signal generator, apply a small input signal to the base of the transistor. With an oscilloscope, compare the input and output signals.

   Require the students to note their observations.

   The students should calculate the gain of the amplifier and observe that the input and output signals are out of phase by 180°.

5. Build the circuit shown below, and monitor the current and voltage as R_2 is adjusted.

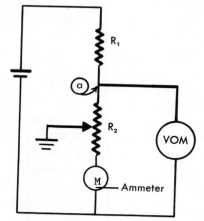

As the R_2 wiper arm is moved upward, the current decreases and the voltage at *a* increases. As the R_2 wiper arm is moved downward, the current increases and the voltage at *a* decreases.

6. Build the operational amplifier circuit shown in Fig. 13-15. Substitute an assortment of electronic components in positions *a* and *b* to demonstrate a number of mathematical operations that can be performed.

PRACTICE PROBLEMS and STUDY QUESTIONS

1. What is the gain of an amplifier if an output signal of 10 V is produced by an input voltage of 10 mV?
2. Voltage and current measurements taken on an operating vacuum tube triode showed that, with a control grid bias of -15 V, the plate current was 100 mA and the plate voltage was 200 V. When the grid bias was changed to -30 V, the plate voltage increased to 310 V and the plate current remained unchanged at 100 mA.
   a. Calculate the gain of this triode.
   b. Calculate the effective resistance (plate resistance) of the triode when the control grid is at:
      (1) -15 V
      (2) -30 V
3. An NPN transistor has a bias voltage of -10 V on the base. An input sine wave with a peak-to-peak amplitude of 10 V is applied to the base. The output voltage taken at the collector has a peak amplitude of 500 V. Calculate the gain of this NPN transistor.
4. Refer to Fig. 13-14.
   Calculate the gain of this operational amplifier when:
   a. $R_1 = 10\ \Omega$ and $R_2 = 100\ k\Omega$
   b. $R_1 = 10\ \Omega$ and $R_2 = 10\ k\Omega$
   c. $R_1 = 5\ \Omega$ and $R_2 = 250\ k\Omega$

ANSWERS
1. 1000
2. a. 7.3
   b. (1) 2 kΩ
      (2) 3.1 kΩ
3. 100
4. a. 10^4
   b. 10^3
   c. 5×10^4

APPROACH TO SOLVING PROBLEMS
1. Gain $= V_{out}/V_{in} = 10$ V/0.01 V $= 1000$
2. a. Gain $= \Delta V_{out}/\Delta V_{in} = 110$ V/15 V $= 7.3$
   b. (1) R $= E/I = 200$ V/100 mA $= 2$ kΩ
      (2) R $= E/I = 310$ V/100 mA $= 3.1$ kΩ
3. Gain $= V_{out}/V_{in} = 500$ V/5 V $= 100$
4. a. Gain $= R_2/R_1 = 100$ kΩ/10 $\Omega = 10^4$
   b. Gain $= R_2/R_1 = 10$ kΩ/10 $\Omega = 10^3$
   c. Gain $= R_2/R_1 = 250$ kΩ/ 5 $\Omega = 5 \times 10^4$

CHAPTER 14

READOUT DEVICES

Readout devices used in clinical laboratory instruments have become increasingly sophisticated with the increased complexity of instruments. However, all readout systems serve the same ultimate function—to supply the operator with required data in correct, clear, and understandable form.

Signal detection and processing have been discussed in earlier chapters. A physical or chemical property of a sample under analysis is detected by a transducer that converts the physical property into an electrical signal. This signal is processed, which usually includes amplification, and is then presented to the readout device. It is important to note that there is a proportionality between the concentration of the detected sample component and the generated electrical signal. Thus the electrical signal can be related to the concentration of a component. This relationship is established when an instrument is calibrated in units of concentration, transmittance, or absorbance or in arbitrarily selected units. A readout device measures the amount of current or voltage generated by a detection system, which in turn presents wanted information about the sample being analyzed.

Commonly used instrument readout (or display) devices to be discussed include meters, recorders, digital displays, and oscilloscopes.

METERS

Housed within a case are the meter face and the meter movement. The meter face displays a scale of units appropriate for the use of that particular meter. The meter movement is a mechanism that deflects from a preset position when current is applied. The degree of deflection is related to the amount of current flowing through the meter movement. The operation of most meter movements used in clinical laboratory instruments is based upon the electromagnetic theory.

The electromagnetic theory as it applies to meter movements can be understood easily with the application of the three basic concepts listed below:

1. When a current flows through a coiled wire, the magnetic lines of force around each loop are concentrated in the center of the coil. These magnetic lines of force form closed loops traveling south to north inside the coil and north to south outside the coil (Fig. 14-1).

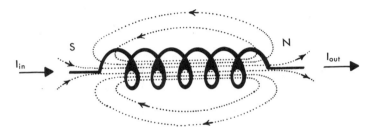

Fig. 14-1. Magnetic field around conducting coil.

2. With increased current flow through the coil, the strength of the magnetic field is increased.

3. Like magnetic poles repel, and unlike magnetic poles attract.

The interaction of the poles of a permanent magnetic field with those of an electromagnetic field is the basis for current measuring devices. A current measuring device, called an *ammeter*, consists of a coiled wire positioned between the poles of a permanent magnet. The orientation of the coiled wire is such that the electromagnetic poles generated by a current are close to their corresponding poles on the permanent magnet. Thus, when a current flows through the coiled wire, the like poles will repel and the coil will deflect or rotate. A coiled spring is attached to the coiled wire assembly to control its degree of deflection and to return it to its original position once current no longer flows through the coiled wire. This permanent magnet–moving coil assembly operates on the principle of D'Arsonval, or moving coil movement, which is the most commonly used movement in clinical laboratory instruments with meter readouts. The original D'Arsonval moving coil movement is used in the galvanometer. The D'Arsonval meter movement is a modification of the D'Arsonval moving coil movement. Both types will be described, since both are still in clinical laboratory instruments.

A galvanometer is a device capable of detecting very small amounts of current. The assembly consists of a permanent magnet and a delicately suspended moving element, of which the degree of rotation is controlled by a very flexible current-carrying spiral spring. The moving element consists of a fine wire wound around a lightweight nonconducting material upon which is mounted a small mirror.

Illustrated in Figs. 14-2 and 14-3, respectively, are the galvanometer moving element assembly and the galvanometer optical arrangement for readout display. Refer to these two figures, and follow the description of how the galvanometer operates. A current generated by a detector is presented to the galvanometer. As the current flows through the suspension wire, the coil, and the spring, a magnetic field is generated around the coil. The polarity of the generated magnetic field is such that its north pole is near the permanent magnet's north pole and its south pole is near the permanent magnet's south pole. The like poles repel each other, and the moving element assembly rotates. A light beam is focused onto the mirror attached to the moving assembly. The light reflected from the mirror is directed to a translucent readout scale. A hairline on the focusing lens is used to indicate

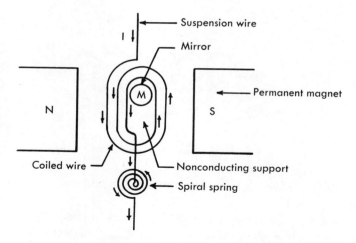

Fig. 14-2. D'Arsonval galvanometer.

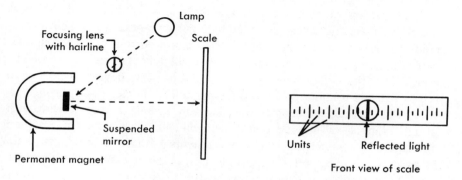

Fig. 14-3. Galvanometer optical arrangement.

the readout point on the scale. As the moving assembly rotates, the reflected light from the mirror moves across the readout scale. When the current through the coil stops, the electromagnetic field around the coil collapses and the moving assembly is returned to its initial or zero position by the spiral spring.

The "zero adjust" on the galvanometer is a delicate adjustment of the spiral spring tension to be made only when no current is flowing through the coil. The zero adjustment can be used to position the reflected image in the center of the readout scale. Using a galvanometer adjusted in this way, current flow through the coil in either direction can be detected and measured. The readout light image will deflect in one direction when current flows in one direction and in the opposite direction when current flows in the other direction. When no current is flowing and the light image is at the preset mid-scale, the image is said to be in the null position.

The high degree of sensitivity of the galvanometer is contributed to by the very lightweight moving coil assembly suspended by the fine phosphor bronze wire and the highly flexible spiral spring. This delicate suspension requires only

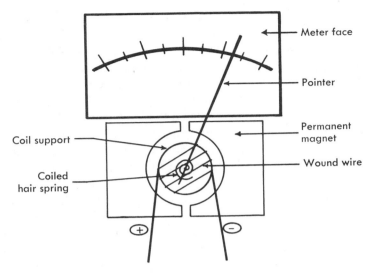

Fig. 14-4. D'Arsonval meter movement.

a very small magnetic force to produce a deflection. The delicacy of construction contributes to the galvanometer's sensitivity; however, it also contributes to its susceptibility to damage from small mechanical shocks. Therefore, a galvanometer should be handled carefully to avoid any physical trauma. Some galvanometers found in spectrophotometers and osmometers consist of moving element assemblies with sturdier suspension to diminish the danger of mechanical damage. Although diminished, the chance of mechanical damage still exists and should be considered when relocating or moving instruments with galvanometer readouts.

The D'Arsonval meter movement is a modified galvanometer. It is not as sensitive as the galvanometer, since the movement assembly is heavier and is mounted on bearings that contribute to the friction to be overcome. Therefore, the meter movement requires more current to generate an electromagnetic field of sufficient strength to rotate the element. The D'Arsonval meter movement is used in instruments in which the amount of current to be measured does not require the high degree of sensitivity provided by the delicate suspension of the D'Arsonval galvanometer. The operation of the meter movement is based upon the same principle as the moving coil movement. The degree of deflection of the movement element assembly depends upon the amount of current flowing through the wire coiled on the element.

As shown in Fig. 14-4, the meter movement assembly is positioned between the curved magnetic poles of a permanent magnet. Linearity of the meter movement rotation is achieved using this arrangement. Magnetic force of repulsion between like magnetic poles is exerted consistently upon the moving element. Thus, the degree of element deflection is directly proportional to the amount of current flowing through the movement assembly.

The meter movement assembly consists of a coil of fine wire wound onto a support fitted with hardened-steel pivots and mounted on jeweled bearings. The jeweled bearing mounting allows the moving element to rotate with a minimum of friction. A pointer attached to the moving assembly deflects across the meter face as the moving element rotates. Matched coiled hair springs are attached above and below the coil assembly to control its degree of rotation and its return to a fixed reference point when there is no current flow. The springs are mounted so that they exert opposing forces on the moving assembly. This arrangement of opposing springs compensates for changes in the spring tension caused by thermal effects. In other words, the expansion or the contraction of one spring because of a temperature change is corrected by the identical change occurring in the opposing spring.

Meter movement damage can result from mechanical shock and/or excess current. Mechanical shock may disrupt the jeweled bearing mounting, thus hindering the smooth rotation of the movement element. Excess current applied to the meter movement may produce a large electromagnetic force, resulting in a rotation of the movement assembly beyond the limit of the control springs. This would stretch and, therefore, ruin the control function of these coiled springs.

D'Arsonval meter movements are used to measure current, voltage, and resistance, which may be displayed on the readout in units of current, voltage, and resistance or in units of other measurements, such as absorbance, transmittance, and concentration. Regardless of the units displayed on the readout scale, the meter is responding to current. It is important to note that the D'Arsonval meter movement is a current measuring device that can be used to relate current to a variety of other parameters. When this meter is used to measure current in a circuit, the meter must be connected in series, as shown in Fig. 14-5. A series arrangement is required in order that the total current in the circuit will flow through the meter and be registered on the meter's readout. An essential characteristic of a current meter is that it have a very small input resistance so that the meter itself does not add an additional resistance to the circuit and therefore change the current. It is important that the measuring device does not alter the value it is measuring.

If the meter is used to measure a potential difference or voltage in a circuit, a meter with a very high input resistance must be connected in parallel across the

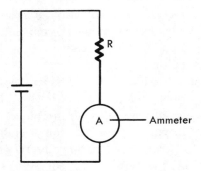

Fig. 14-5. Series connection of ammeter in circuit.

two points between which the potential difference is to be measured. This arrangement is shown in Fig. 14-6. As illustrated in this figure, if the potential difference between points *a* and *b* is to be determined, a voltmeter must be connected in parallel to R_1. This parallel arrangement allows for voltage measurement with minimal effect on the current flow in the circuit. The required high input resistance will prevent an appreciable current drain from the circuit. A current drain would result in the undesirable situation of the measuring device altering the value to be measured.

All meter movements have an internal resistance resulting from the resistance of the current-carrying elements. The factors of length, cross sectional diameter, and resistivity of the wire used in the construction of the coil are used to calculate the internal resistance, which is indicated on the meter face or in the specifications of the meter. Since each meter has a fixed internal resistance, Ohm's law ($E = IR$) can be applied to measure the voltage across the meter through its direct relationship to current. In this way, a current meter can be used for voltage measurement.

The amount of current required to deflect a meter movement full-scale is referred to as the sensitivity of the meter. The smaller the current required for full-scale deflection, the greater the meter's sensitivity. Sensitivity depends upon two construction characteristics of the meter. First, the greater the number of turns in the coil, the smaller the amount of current required to generate an electromagnetic field strong enough to deflect the coil assembly. Second, the weight of the assembly, the friction of the bearings, and the tension of the controlling hair springs influence the amount of energy required for coil rotation. Meter sensitivity using current is expressed in amps, milliamps, or microamps. The lower the current, the higher the meter sensitivity.

Although sensitivity, in its strictest definition, is the amount of current required to produce full-scale deflection, this term is also related to meter voltage drop and meter internal resistance. Meter voltage drop, usually given in millivolts, is the amount of voltage dropped across the internal resistance when full-scale deflection current is flowing. Ohms-per-volt is another expression of meter sensitivity. This value is calculated by dividing the meter internal resistance by the

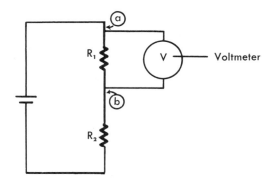

Fig. 14-6. Parallel connection of voltmeter in circuit.

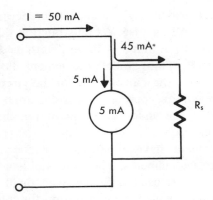

Fig. 14-7. Range extension of ammeter.

full-scale voltage. The higher the ohms-per-volt ratio, the less current required for full-scale deflection, and thus the more sensitive the meter. The ohms-per-volt value is frequently indicated on the meter face.

Design and construction of a meter determine sensitivity and, therefore, the range in which a particular meter can be used. Meters with only one range are of limited use. For example, a meter with an internal resistance (R_m) of 100 Ω and a sensitivity of 5 mA can be used to measure currents of no more than 5 mA and voltages of no more than:

$$E = IR = (5 \text{ mA})(100 \text{ }\Omega) = 500 \text{ mV}$$

Fortunately, the limitation of the fixed range of a meter movement can be eliminated by connecting resistors in series or parallel to the meter. The circuit configuration used depends upon the use of the meter. If the meter is used as an ammeter, the resistors are connected in parallel to the meter movement. A voltmeter's range is extended by connecting the resistors in series with the meter movement.

The methods of extending the ranges of an ammeter and a voltmeter are demonstrated in the following example.

An available meter has an internal resistance of 100 Ω, a sensitivity of 5 mA, and a full-scale voltage of 500 mV. This meter must be used to measure currents up to 50 mA and voltages up to 50 V.

Fig. 14-7 illustrates the addition of a resistor to extend the range of the meter when it is to be used as an ammeter. The resistor is connected in parallel to divert or shunt from the meter the current in excess of 5 mA. Since the range is to be extended to 50 mA, 45 mA must be shunted around the meter. From the concept of current division, it is evident that the shunt resistor (R_s) can be selected with a value appropriate for diverting 45 mA through the shunt. The voltage drop across the meter is the same as that across the parallel shunt — 500 mV. The shunt resistor value is calculated as shown below.

$$R_s = E_{fs}/I_s$$

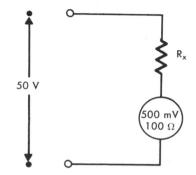

Fig. 14-8. Range extension of voltmeter.

where:

R_s = Value of shunt resistor
E_{fs} = Full-scale deflection voltage
I_s = Current through the shunt

R_s = 500 mV/45 mA = 11.11 Ω

Illustrated in Fig. 14-8 is the range extension of the meter when used as a voltmeter. In accordance with the principle of voltage division, the resistor R_x (known as the "multiplier") is connected in series with the meter so as to drop voltage in excess of 500 mV (the full-scale voltage). Since 50 V is to be measured with this meter, 49.5 V must be dropped across R_x. To determine the value of R_x, first calculate the total resistance required for a circuit with a voltage of 50 V and a current of 5 mA, and then subtract the meter resistance as shown below.

R_T = E/I = 50 V/5 mA = 10,000 Ω
R_x = R_T − R_m
R_x = 10,000 Ω − 100 Ω = 9,900 Ω

RECORDERS

Recorders are readout devices used almost as much as meters in clinical laboratory instruments. Functionally, meters and recorders are the same—that is, a signal produced by the detector and processed by the signal processing unit is displayed in a form of understandable data. The advantage recorders have over meters is that the display data are presented as a permanent record.

Two major classifications of recorders are the moving coil or galvanometer recorders and the potentiometric recorders. The potentiometric recorders are most commonly used in the clinical laboratory. However, both types will be discussed, the moving coil recorder briefly and the potentiometric recorder in more detail.

The electromagnetic principle upon which the operation of moving coil meters is based is also applicable to moving coil or galvanometer recorders. An electromagnetic field is generated by a current passing through a conducting coiled wire on a moving coil assembly. The assembly mounted between the poles of a permanent magnet is rotated as the electromagnetic and permanent magnetic fields interact. The degree of rotation is proportional to the strength of the electromagnetic field, which is in turn related to the amount of current flowing through the coiled wire. Rotation of the assembly is recorded by some type of transcribing device. These devices are of two types, indirect writing and direct writing. The type of indicator attached to the moving coil assembly determines whether a moving coil or galvanometer recorder is indirect or direct writing.

In both types of recorders, chart paper is the permanent record. A chart drive moves at a constant rate the chart paper upon which the indicator element traces the output data. Thus the final recorded data is presented on a time axis.

The indicator element on an indirect writing recorder can be a reflected light beam or an ink jet. Recorders using the reflected light beam are called oscillographic recorders. The moving coil assembly is similar to that of the D'Arsonval galvanometer, with a mirror attached to the moving coil. The reflected light beam is focused onto photosensitive chart paper, producing a chart tracing. This type of optical recorder has a very high frequency response of above 150 Hz and as high as 4.8 kHz. That is, this type of recorder is capable of recording signals presented to it at a rate above 150 signals per second. This frequency response is possible because the moving coil assembly, like that in the galvanometer, with its extremely low inertia, responds to very small amounts of current.

A disadvantage of the oscillographic recorder is that the chart tracing must be developed in a darkroom. To eliminate the need for photographic development, oscillographic recorders have been introduced in which ultraviolet light replaces the visible light source. The ultraviolet light beam is focused onto a self-developing chart paper that produces the permanent tracing.

The other type of indirect writing recorder uses an ink jet expelled from a capillary onto the moving chart paper. The inertia of this moving coil assembly is slightly greater than that of the optical recorders. However, the frequency response of the ink jet recorder is as high as 1 kHz.

The direct writing moving coil recorders are classified as medium frequency recorders. They respond to frequencies up to a maximum of 105 Hz. Direct writing recorders are available with an ink pen or a heated stylus attached to the moving coil assembly. The ink pen type uses untreated chart paper upon which the ink flows by capillary action to produce a permanent chart tracing. Heat-sensitive paper is used in the heated stylus type. The heated stylus produces a tracing on the heat-sensitive chart paper.

The most commonly used recorder in the clinical laboratory is the potentiometric recorder. This type of recorder is classified as a low-frequency recorder, responding to signals from 0 to approximately 5 Hz. The potentiometric recorder utilizes a null-balancing measuring system, illustrated in a simplified block diagram in Fig. 14-9. The input voltage is from an analytical instrument, for example, a spectrophotometer. The reference voltage is a constant voltage source supplied by a mercury cell or generated by the power supply within the circuit. The difference between the input voltage (V_{in}) and the reference voltage (V_{ref}) is called the error voltage (V_{error}):

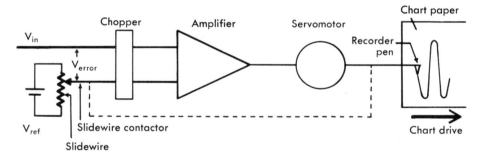

Fig. 14-9. Simplified block diagram of null-balancing potentiometric recorder.

$$V_{in} - V_{ref} = V_{error}$$

The input voltage and reference voltage are compared, and the error voltage is converted by a chopper (a device that permits intermittent passage of two signals that are to be compared to each other) to a pulsating dc signal, which is then amplified, usually by an operational amplifier. The amplified error voltage drives a servomotor (*servo* is Latin for slave; the servomotor is a slave to the error voltage). The greater the error voltage, the faster the servomotor rotates. A smaller error voltage drives the servomotor more slowly, and an error voltage of zero provides no force to the servomotor, and the servomotor stops. The servomotor is mechanically connected to both the slide wire contactor and the recorder pen, as is indicated by the dashed line in Fig. 14-9. The servomotor drives the pen and the slide wire contactor simultaneously. The slide wire offers a resistance over which the reference voltage is dropped—that is, it is a variable resistor or potentiometer. Therefore, as the slide wire contactor is moved along the slide wire, the reference voltage provided to the circuit is altered. As the servomotor drives the slide wire contactor, the reference voltage is continuously changed and compared to the input voltage. Once the slide wire contactor reaches the null position (where the reference voltage equals the input voltage), the error voltage is zero and the servomotor stops, as do the recorder pen and the slide wire contactor on the reference potentiometer. The servomotor does not operate again until a different input voltage is applied. This rebalancing is continuous and begins immediately with any change in input voltage.

Three adjustments on potentiometric recorders to be considered are the range, the zero, and the gain adjustments. These three adjustments are indicated in Fig. 14-10. The potentiometric reference circuit is more detailed than the one shown in Fig. 14-9. Since the complexity of actual recorder circuits can be confusing, overly simplified diagrams are used to present potentiometric recorder operational principles.

The range of a recorder may be indicated, for example, as 1 mV. This means that full deflection of the pen across the graph paper is equal to an input voltage of 1 mV. Thus, 10 mV and 100 mV ranges mean that full deflection of the pen is caused by the input voltages of 10 mV and 100 mV, respectively. As is in-

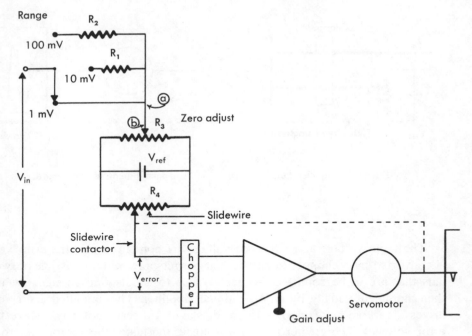

Fig. 14-10. Null-balancing potentiometric recorder.

dicated in Fig. 14-10, the range is determined by introducing resistances over which the input voltage will be dropped to a maximum value of 1 mV at point *a*. For example, in the 10 mV range, if 10 mV is the input voltage, the value of R_1 is such that there is a 9 mV voltage drop across this resistor. Therefore, point *a* is at 1 mV, and the circuit functions as if the 1 mV range were being used. The same is true for the 100 mV range. When 100 mV is the input voltage, the voltage drop over R_2 is 99 mV; therefore, point *a* is at 1 mV.

The range of a recorder may be specifically indicated, as described above, or selected from a continuous scale from 1 to 100 mV. In the latter case, the range selector could be a variable resistor as shown in Fig. 14-11 instead of a set of fixed resistors as indicated in Fig. 14-10. The variable resistor type of range selector is needed when full deflection of the pen must be set on the chart paper. For example, when using a recording spectrophotometer, the operator sets the pen at full deflection (100% transmittance) when the blank is read for a procedure using a direct color reaction, such as the procedure for determining the concentration of blood urea nitrogen (BUN). The recorder is being "told" (calibrated) that this is the maximum voltage to be recorded throughout the procedure.

The "zero adjust" is used to set the recorder pen at a baseline. In essence, the recorder is being "told" the value of the minimum voltage to be applied during a procedure. In a BUN colorimetric procedure using a recording spectrophotometer, all the light is blocked from the photodetector. Even though no light is hitting the photodetector, a small amount of current will flow in the circuit because of free electrons thermally liberated from the photodetector. This current

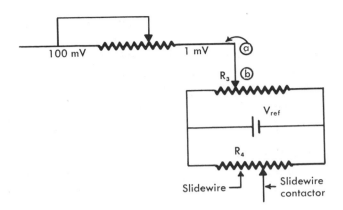

Fig. 14-11. Variable resistor range selector.

is called dark current. The dark current voltage is eliminated from the circuit by dropping it across a variable resistor, R_3 (Fig. 14-10). The contactor B on R_3 is adjusted until the pen reads zero on the chart paper.

The "gain adjust" controls signal amplification. The higher the gain of the amplifier, the greater the resulting signal amplification. Thus the amplifier increases the error signal to a level that will drive the servomotor. If the gain, or amplification, is reduced, the amount of error signal needed to move the pen will be larger. If the gain is increased, the amount of error signal needed to move the pen will be smaller.

The gain adjust is conceptually shown in Fig. 14-10. This control is used to increase or decrease the response of the servomotor to the error voltage. If the gain is too high, the pen will respond to such a small signal change that it will chatter, or oscillate back and forth, even though no apparent input signal is received. This is called "noise." The gain must be reduced until the noise stops. On the other hand, if the gain is too low, the pen will respond sluggishly or not at all to input signals.

In most potentiometric recorders, the chart is driven at a constant rate by a motor drive. This produces a linear time axis. Time (T) is one axis, and a variable (Y) is the other. These recorders are called T-Y recorders or, more commonly, "stripchart" recorders.

The stripchart potentiometric recorder has been modified to produce two other types of potentiometric recorders, the X-Y recorder and the linear-logarithmic recorder. The modification was the addition of another set of slide wires and servomotor. Since these potentiometric recorders are not commonly used in the clinical laboratory, they will be described only briefly.

The X-Y recorder has two sets of slide wire and servomotor systems. One of these systems moves the pen along the X-axis (abcissa), while the other system moves it along the Y-axis (ordinate). Plotted on a chart are two variables, neither of which is time. In some X-Y recorders the chart moves (usually on the X-axis), and one of the variables can be recorded in relation to time — that is, the variable has a time base. A stripchart recorder may be used to plot enzyme activity against time, but an X-Y recorder can provide more information by plotting, for example, enzyme activity against temperature change. In this example, one of the X-Y recorder systems would be detecting enzymatic change while the other system would be monitoring temperature change over time.

The linear-logarithmic recorder contains two separate sets of slide wires and amplifiers. One set is a linear amplifier and slide wire used for plotting data in linear form. Data can be plotted in logarithmic form by using the logarithmic amplifier and slide wire.

Three important recorder characteristics in addition to frequency response, described earlier in this chapter, are chart speed, pen response, and sensitivity. Chart speed is the rate at which the chart paper moves, usually expressed in inches or centimeters per minute. Pen response is the time (in seconds or milliseconds) required for the pen to move from one edge of the chart paper to the other when full-scale voltage is applied. Recorder sensitivity is a measurement of the degree of deflection caused by a unit of current and is expressed in centimeters per microampere or milliampere.

The graphic presentation of recorders is a series of peaks on a chart. The concentration of a constituent of an analyzed sample can be determined by relating concentration to either the height of a peak or the area under a peak. Relating peak height to concentration presents no particular problems and can be done very easily. However, relating the area under the peak to concentration presents the problem of determining the area under the peak, the process called integration. If the graph paper used is divided into very small squares, the squares under each peak could be counted to determine the area. This method is not ideal. It is tedious, time consuming, and subject to inaccuracy resulting from human error. Integration of peaks has been automated by incorporating an integrator into recorders used for applications requiring peak integrations—for example, in densitometers used to quantify protein fractions separated by protein electrophoresis.

Integrators are of two types, mechanical and electronic. The mechanical integrator consists of a disc rotated at a constant rate. Upon the disc is a freely rotating ball. The rate at which the ball rotates is determined by its position on the rotating disc. If it is at the center of the disc, it does not rotate. Near the center it rotates slowly, and at the edge of the disc it rotates very rapidly. The ball is contained within a small assembly that supports two separate mechanical linkages to two separate pens, the recorder pen and an integrator pen that is positioned at the edge of the graph paper. The movement of the recorder pen determines the position of the ball on the rotating disc. When the recorder pen is at zero, the ball is in the center of the disc, and when the recorder pen is at maximum deflection, the ball is on the edge of the rotating disc. The integrator pen responds to the rate at which the ball rotates. With each rotation or with a specified number of rotations (depending upon the design of the integrator), the pen makes a stroke along the edge of the graph paper. Therefore, the greater the area under the peak, the more integration strokes will be made. Since the number of integration strokes is directly related to the area under the peak, the number of strokes can be related to sample constituent concentration.

Electronic integrators are replacing the mechanical type. Various types of electronic integrators are available. One type consists of accurate capacitors that are used to store a small fraction of the signal driving the recorder pen. Once the capacitor is charged to a certain potential, it is discharged, causing an integrator pen to produce a stroke on the edge of the chart paper. Another type of electronic integrator uses an operational amplifier to generate the data representative of the · area under the peaks.

DIGITAL DISPLAYS

In clinical laboratory instruments, digital readouts are in the process of replacing conventional meters containing meter movements. This new generation of readouts is capable of displaying information in alphabetic or numeric form. Analog-to-digital conversion occurs within the digital circuitry, which changes electrical signals to digital binary form that is then converted to decimal arithmetic numbers. Digital displays require associated electronic circuitry to accept input information and apply required voltages to the appropriate readout elements. This associated circuitry is called the drive circuitry of the readout display device.

Digital readouts have several advantages over conventional meters. They are not susceptible to mechanical shock as the meter movement assemblies are. Digital display systems are more accurate than meters. Data presented in digital form eliminates possible reading error caused by parallax. (Parallax is an optical illusion that makes an object appear displaced when viewed from an angle. Thus a meter pointer's position on a readout scale depends upon the angle from which it is read. To eliminate such errors, the eye should be aligned directly above the meter pointer.)

Brief descriptions of common types of digital displays will be presented. Two broad classifications of digital readout systems are electromechanical and electronic. Electromechanical readouts used in clinical laboratory instruments are the coupled-wheel or drum type. This mechanical register consists of a number of wheels coupled in such a way that each can be rotated independently. Rotation of the wheels is caused by the driving force from the servomotor or electronic source. Upon each wheel are printed the digits 0 through 9. Thus, rotation of the coupled wheels can display numeric data containing a number of digits equal to the number of wheels in the electromechanical readout device.

Electromechanical readout devices have a maximum frequency of approximately 15 to 20 Hz. This low frequency response limits the use of this type of readout to those analytical instruments for which high frequency response is not required. For example, these readouts could not be used in particle counters, since rapid response to particle-produced signals and immediate digital display are required. An application for which mechanical registers commonly have been used is readouts in emission flame photometers. The continuous signals generated in this instrument are compatible with the response of the mechanical readout. This type of readout is not susceptible to damage by mechanical jarring or vibration. It is also inexpensive and operated by simple electronic circuitry. Therefore, replacement of mechanical with electronic displays in clinical laboratory instruments (for example, flame photometers) was not initiated by the limitations of mechanical registers but rather by the popularity of electronic displays.

Electronic readouts are the most popular of digital readout displays. The first to be developed was the NIXIE tube, followed by the filament segment tube. With the surge of advances in solid-state electronics, two types of solid-state displays have evolved, the light-emitting diode (LED) and the planar glow panel.

The NIXIE tube consists of a glass tube containing neon gas and a maximum of 12 stacked filaments in the form of numbers or letters. A specific number or letter is illuminated when a potential of 100 to 180 V is applied to that alphabetic or numeric filament. Although the operating voltage is high, the driving circuitry is relatively simple when compared to that of other electronic readout displays.

In the filament segment tube, the operating voltage is decreased to 15 to 25 V, while the complexity of the driving circuitry is increased. The segmented type of display, shown in Fig. 14-12, consists of seven filaments that can be selectively illuminated for an alphabetic or numeric display.

The solid-state light emitting diode (LED) type of digital display is available as a seven-segmented display or as a 36-diode X-Y array readout. The diodes used in these readout devices are the gallium arsenide type. The advantage of this display over the earlier ones is its very low power consumption. It requires an operating voltage of 1.75 V with a current of 50 mA. The seven-segmented display consists of seven rod-shaped diodes in the configuration shown in Fig. 14-12.

The other type of LED display consists of small dot-shaped diodes arranged as illustrated in Fig. 14-13. Alphanumeric characters are displayed with the selective illumination of the diodes in the array. Only 5 to 10 mA current is required to illuminate one character in this display.

Planar glow panel or planar panel solid-state displays consist of double-anode, single-cathode gas discharge diodes arranged in an 111-dot X-Y array. The diode anodes are oriented with one of the anodes toward the front of the panel and the other toward the back. When a dot in the array is to be visible on the panel, its front anode is illuminated. Those dots not visible on the panel are diodes with their back anodes illuminated. Thus, alphanumeric characters are displayed with the illumination of the anode positioned in the front panel of the array.

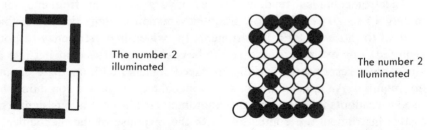

The number 2 illuminated

The number 2 illuminated

Fig. 14-12. Seven segment display.   **Fig. 14-13.** X-Y array of light-emitting diodes.

OSCILLOSCOPES OR CATHODE RAY TUBES (CRT)

The oscilloscope is a readout device used for viewing electrical waveforms; measuring voltage, current, and frequency; and determining phase relationships between signals. Another name for the oscilloscope is cathode ray tube (CRT). CRTs are included in clinical laboratory instruments when the visualization of electrical signals is required in monitoring sample analyses. For example, most electronic particle counters have a CRT upon which are displayed the electrical impulses produced by individual particles. The final particle counts are presented on digital readout displays.

Oscilloscopes are used to measure electrical signal parameters. To measure voltage, an operator first calibrates the oscilloscope by observing on the screen the amplitude of a known voltage. The unknown voltage is then determined by comparing its amplitude to that of the known voltage, since the ratio of amplitudes is equal to the ratio of the voltages. Current in a circuit is calculated by measuring the voltage drop across a known resistance in the circuit. To determine the frequency of a signal, the operator first calibrates the CRT screen with a signal of known frequency. The unknown frequency of the signal can then be measured on the calibrated screen of the CRT.

The cathode ray tube consists of three major parts enclosed in an evacuated tube: an electron gun, two sets of deflection plates, and a screen (Fig. 14-14). The electron gun generates a well-focused electron beam. The gun consists of a heated cathode, a control grid, a focusing anode, and an accelerating anode. Free electrons are emitted from the hot cathode. An aperture in the control grid allows a small stream of electrons to pass. The potential of the control grid is negative with respect to the cathode and therefore functions as the control grid in the vacuum tube triode functions—that is, to control the number of electrons passing through. The electron beam intensity is controlled by adjusting the potential on the control grid. The focusing anode is the first anode beyond the control grid. The potential of the focusing anode is very positive with respect to the cathode. Thus the

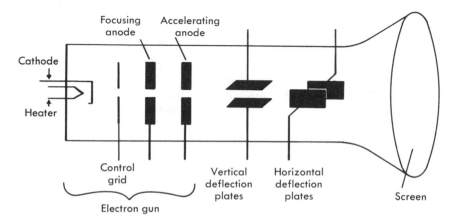

Fig. 14-14. Cathode ray tube.

electrons are accelerated and the beam is concentrated as it passes through the anode's aperture. Adjustment of the potential on this anode controls the sharpness of the electron beam. A more positive potential on the next anode, the accelerating anode, increasingly accelerates electron flow. The electron beam produced by the electron gun is directed to the center of the screen.

Before reaching the screen, the electron beam passes through two pairs of parallel plates, the horizontal and vertical deflection plates, oriented at right angles to each other. One of each of the two sets of plates is maintained at a fixed potential, usually equal to the potential on the accelerating anode. When the other plate of a set is made positive, the electron beam is attracted toward that plate. Therefore, a positive potential applied to the variable plate of the horizontal or vertical deflection plates causes the electron beam to be deflected horizontally or vertically. Deflection in the opposite direction is obtained with the application of a negative potential to the variable plate with respect to the fixed plate. The negative potential repels the electron beam. With application of voltages to both the vertical and horizontal deflection plates simultaneously, the electron beam can be deflected in any direction. The direction and extent of deflection depends on the relative magnitudes of the two voltages.

The interior surface of the screen is coated with a fluorescent or phosphorescent material that emits visible light when its molecules are bombarded by electrons. Thus, the deflections of the electron beam produce a highly visible trace on the CRT.

One of the associated circuits of the oscilloscope is a time base generator that applies a sawtooth voltage signal to the horizontal deflection plate. This causes the electron beam to move at a constant rate across the screen and then return rapidly to the starting position to begin another sweep across the screen. In this way, the signal displayed on a CRT is the voltage change with respect to time.

INSTRUCTIONAL ACTIVITIES

1. Display different readout devices, for example, galvanometer, meter movement, electromechanical register, electronic readout displays, and oscilloscope.
2. Require that students identify and describe the operation of readouts utilized in analytical instruments they have used in their biological, chemical, and physical science laboratories.
3. Demonstrate the use of meters, recorders, and oscilloscopes while discussing the operation and function of each control adjustment.
4. Using a sensitive ammeter, extend its range for use as an ammeter and as a voltmeter so that several ranges are available for each mode of operation.

PRACTICE PROBLEMS and STUDY QUESTIONS

1. An ammeter has an internal resistance of 100 Ω and a full-scale deflection with 10 mA. Calculate and indicate the values of all components in circuit diagrams illustrating the extension of the meter range to:
   a. 1 A
   b. 10 V
2. Volts are dropped across a meter movement when 20 mA maximally deflects the meter pointer. Draw a circuit diagram indicating how the range of this meter could be extended to 100 V. Calculate and indicate the values of all components in the circuit diagram.
3. Referring to the multiple range ammeter shown below, calculate the resistances for the shunt resistors: $R_{s}1$, $R_{s}2$, $R_{s}3$, and $R_{s}4$.

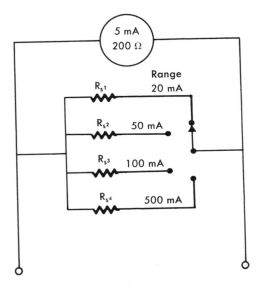

4. Referring to the multiple range voltmeter shown below, calculate the resistances for the multiplier resistors $R_{x}1$, $R_{x}2$, $R_{x}3$, and $R_{x}4$.

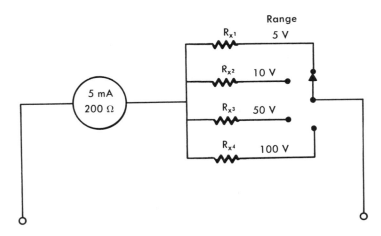

ANSWERS
1. a.

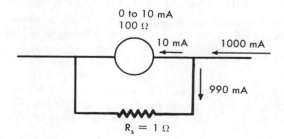

0 to 10 mA
100 Ω

10 mA   1000 mA

990 mA

$R_s = 1\ \Omega$

b.

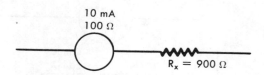

10 mA
100 Ω

$R_x = 900\ \Omega$

2.

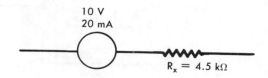

10 V
20 mA

$R_x = 4.5\ k\Omega$

3.   20 mA range: $R_{s1} = 66.67\ \Omega$
     50 mA range: $R_{s2} = 22.22\ \Omega$
   100 mA range: $R_{s3} = 10.53\ \Omega$
   500 mA range: $R_{s4} = 2.02\ \Omega$

4.   5 V range: $R_{x1} = 0.8\ k\Omega$
   10 V range: $R_{x2} = 1.8\ k\Omega$
   50 V range: $R_{x3} = 9.8\ k\Omega$
  100 V range: $R_{x4} = 19.8\ k\Omega$

APPROACH TO SOLVING PROBLEMS

1. a. $R_s = E_{fs}/I_s$
     $R_s = (IR)_m/I_s = (1\ V)/990\ mA = 1\ \Omega$
  b. $R_T = E/I = 10\ V/0.01\ A = 1\ k\Omega$
     $R_x = R_T - R_m = 1000\ \Omega - 100\ \Omega = 900\ \Omega$
2. $R_m = E_{fs}/I_{fs} = 10\ V/20\ mA = 500\ \Omega$
   $R_T = E/I = 100\ V/0.02\ A = 5\ k\Omega$
   $R_x = R_T - R_m = 5\ k\Omega - 0.5\ k\Omega = 4.5\ k\Omega$
3. $E_{fs} = IR = (0.005\ A)(200\ \Omega) = 1\ V$
   20 mA range: $R_s = E_{fs}/I_s = 1\ V/15\ mA = 66.67\ \Omega$
   50 mA range: $R_s = E_{fs}/I_s = 1\ V/45\ mA = 22.22\ \Omega$
  100 mA range: $R_s = E_{fs}/I_s = 1\ V/95\ mA = 10.53\ \Omega$
  500 mA range: $R_s = E_{fs}/I_s = 1\ V/495\ mA = 2.02\ \Omega$
4.   5 V range: $R_T = E/I_{fs} = 5\ V/5\ mA = 1\ k\Omega$
           $R_x = R_T - R_m = 1\ k\Omega - 0.2\ k\Omega = 0.8\ k\Omega$
   10 V range: $R_T = E/I_{fs} = 10\ V/5\ mA = 2\ k\Omega$
           $R_x = R_T - R_m = 2\ k\Omega - 0.2\ k\Omega = 1.8\ k\Omega$
   50 V range: $R_T = E/I_{fs} = 50\ V/5\ mA = 10\ k\Omega$
           $R_x = R_T - R_m = 10\ k\Omega - 0.2\ k\Omega = 9.8\ k\Omega$
  100 V range: $R_T = E/I_{fs} = 100\ V/5\ mA = 20\ k\Omega$
           $R_x = R_T - R_m = 20\ k\Omega - 0.2\ k\Omega = 19.8\ k\Omega$

Safety and troubleshooting

Of primary importance in working with electrical equipment is an appreciation of the possible hazards involved. Safety precautions should be taken at all times in operating or working on electrical devices. Precautions discussed in this section include: recognition of training limitations, adequate grounding, insulation of conductors, self-protection, circuit modifications, and extinguishing electrical fires. Another important aspect of instrumentation discussed in this section is troubleshooting. A general logical approach to troubleshooting is presented.

CHAPTER 15

ELECTRICAL SAFETY

The proliferation of electronic instruments in the clinical laboratory has increased recognition of the hazards associated with their operation. Laboratory personnel should be keenly aware of the danger of electric shock and informed of the precautions to be taken when working with electronic instruments.

ELECTRIC SHOCK

Fortunately, electric shock is not always fatal; however, it is responsible for hundreds of deaths each year. Conduction of an electrical current through human tissue results in the unpleasant sensation called electric shock. Since body fluids contain electrolytes, they are good electrical conductors. Therefore, when the body makes contact between two points of differing potential, it serves as a conducting pathway for current flow.

The severity of a shock is determined by the amount of current and its route of flow through the body. Although body fluids are conductors, the body is provided with a very effective insulation against shock. Dry, unbroken skin is a good insulating material. When the skin is wet, the resistance of the body's insulating covering decreases drastically, altering the body's resistance from the megohm range with dry skin to as low as 300 Ω. Such a change in body resistance affects the magnitude of current produced by the potential applied across the body. For example, if a 60 Hz ac potential of 115 V were applied across the body when the skin is wet, the resulting current could be greater than 300 mA.

The magnitude and the pathway of current passing through the body are influential factors in determining the type and severity of damage inflicted. Current flow is accompanied by heat dissipation, which is responsible for varying degrees of burns. Electrochemical action potentials are the communicating links between the nervous and the muscular systems. Externally introduced electric current may interrupt the electrical impulses of the neuromuscular communicating network or may exert direct effects on muscles to cause contraction. Stimulation of the neuromuscular system with a 1 mA current is felt as a tingling sensation. Currents above 10 mA cause muscle contractions sufficiently severe to result in temporary paralysis. This electrically induced paralysis prevents the

159

release of the grip on the conductor (source of electric shock). Currents passing through vital organs may interfere with their normal functions and result in death. For example, if the muscle-contracting electrical impulses propagated across the heart are altered, ventricular fibrillation and death may result. Thus, if a 60 Hz ac current of 100 mA passes through the body arm-to-arm or arm-to-opposite leg, death is a likely outcome.

The phase "current, not voltage, kills" is significant. When working with electrical devices, operators should take every precaution to prevent current flow through the body. Therefore, the body should never be put into a position to function as a circuit-completing conductor.

ELECTRICAL SAFETY PRECAUTIONS

Safety precautions to be taken in working with electrical instruments are itemized and briefly discussed below. Simply being aware of such precautions is inadequate for effective avoidance of potential electrical hazards: these safety practices must be an integral part of daily routine.

Recognition of training limitations

The most important precaution that can be taken during the operation of electrical instruments is that the operator perform only those functions within his or her capabilities. Understanding Ohms' law and knowing how to use a VOM certainly do not constitute a license to probe irresponsibly into instrument circuits. The repair of electronic malfunctions should be performed only by those who are adequately trained to do so. For example, in a spectrophotometer, changing a blown fuse, a burned out light bulb, or a damaged photovoltaic cell is within the capabilities of all technical laboratory personnel, while replacing a power supply would probably require a qualified electronics technician.

Adequate grounding

Protection against electric shock is the primary function of grounding instruments. Usually the instrument chassis is connected to ground to drain to earth unwanted, dangerous voltage that may collect on the chassis from current leakage or from a short in the circuit. By touching two points, an ungrounded instrument upon which a potential has collected and a conductor to ground (for example, a water pipe), an individual serves as a conductor through which current will flow from the higher potential (the instrument chassis) to ground. The metal chassis of two different instruments may carry different potentials because of their differing degrees of effectiveness of grounding. Therefore, if both instruments were touched at the same time, current would flow hand-to-hand from the higher to the lower potential. For this reason, an instrument and a ground or another instrument should never be touched simultaneously.

Protection by grounding is effective only when a good, continuous ground connection exists. Power cords on most instruments have three-prong plugs. The third (round) prong serves as the connector between the ground lead attached to the instrument chassis and the ground conductor into the earth.

First, the adequacy of the grounding outlet should be determined by a competent electrician.

Second, a continuous ground conducting pathway from the instrument to the grounded outlet should be ensured. Removal of the ground pin on the three-prong plug breaks the grounding circuit, rendering the grounding protection ineffective. Use of "cheater" plugs (two-to-three prong adapters) is essentially the same as removing the grounding pin. The grounding lead on the cheater plug should be connected to a ground, but such ground attachments are not usually reliable. For example, this ground lead is frequently attached to a screw on the outlet receptacle plate, but if the screw is coated with paint (an insulating material) or is not connected directly to ground, such an attachment is of no value, providing only false security. Removing a plug from outlet receptacles by pulling on the cord may break or loosen the ground wire, thus diminishing the effectiveness of the grounding protection. Use of extension cords may also jeopardize grounding protection, in addition to presenting a tripping hazard. If absolutely required, extension cords should be the heavy-duty type with three-prong plugs.

Third, the ground lead should be securely attached to the instrument chassis. This connection must be metal-to-metal to provide a conducting connection. If this lead becomes loose or disconnected, grounding protection is diminished or eliminated. If an instrument is not effectively grounded and the chassis collects a charge, that charge can be transferred to a conductor that comes into contact with it. Therefore, operating instruments should not be placed on metal surfaces such as metal carts or tables.

Insulation of conductors

Conducting leads in an instrument should be insulated. An exposed conducting wire may result in electric shock and/or circuit damage. It should be evident from the earlier discussion of electric shock that if an exposed conducting wire were touched by a person in contact with a ground connection, electric shock would be experienced. A short in a circuit (for example, if an exposed conducting wire makes contact with the instrument chassis) will draw a large amount of current. This current will flow from the power outlet, through the circuit to the shorted connection, and then to ground. If the instrument chassis is not grounded, a large potential will be stored on the chassis. The large current passing through the circuit generates excess heat, which may damage or ruin electronic components.

To avoid electric shock and/or circuit damage caused by exposed conductors, periodically visually inspect the accessible circuit wiring for frayed wires and cracked or melted insulation coatings on electrical leads. Wires with damaged insulation should be replaced immediately. Also, a conscious effort should be made to keep electrical cables and circuit wiring in good condution. Electrical cables should not be stepped on or run over with carts. Cleaning solvents containing alcohol should not be used to clean electrical equipment, since alcohol damages most types of insulation varnishes.

Self-protection

Protective measures taken by an instrument operator may be life saving and therefore should be consistently practiced. The following self-protective practices are essential for electrical safety. Read a new instrument's instruction manual before operating the instrument. Note and observe special operating and maintenance instructions. Report immediately the slightest shock obtained from an instrument. Turn off and unplug instruments before performing repairs.

Do not assume that the circuit of an unplugged and/or turned-off instrument is safe to probe into indiscriminately. The capacitors in the circuit may hold their charge even when the circuit is no longer energized. These capacitors are discharged in circuits designed to include "bleeder" resistors. Bleeder resistors are resistors connected in parallel to capacitors so as to discharge the capacitors to ground when the circuit is turned off. However, if the circuit design is not well understood, it is best to assume that potentials may be stored within the circuit and to approach the circuit as if it were energized.

When working on circuits, follow some key rules. Keep one hand away from conducting surfaces to avoid hand-to-hand electric shock (a lab coat pocket is a safe place for that second hand). Use only insulated tools. Keep work area, hands, and clothes dry. If you are standing on a damp surface (for example, a concrete basement floor), wear rubber soled shoes. Do not wear metal jewelry such as rings, wristwatches, or loose necklaces and bracelets, since a short circuit may result from contact with these conducting ornaments.

Those whose capabilities and training permit them to work on high voltage circuits should not work alone, and assistance should be immediately available if required.

Those whose confidence outweighs their respect for electricity and their common sense should either reevaluate and change their attitudes or seek another pastime.

Circuit modifications

Circuit modifications should be left to the electrical engineer. Components replaced in an instrument should be in compliance with the instrument's specifications. Fuses should be replaced with fuses of specified ratings. Jumpers or other conducting substitutes should not be used to bypass a fuse. The fuse serves to protect the circuit from damage caused by excess current. Therefore, the fuse is an important circuit component that should be used properly.

The blowing of a fuse is a warning of an electronic problem that should be identified and corrected immediately.

Extinguishing electrical fires

The generation of excess heat by high current may cause an electrical fire. If smoke and/or odor indicate burning within a circuit, the instrument should be turned off and unplugged immediately. Carbon dioxide – type fire extinguishers are used on electrical fires. Water and foams are electrical conductors and therefore should not be used on electrical fires.

Poisonous selenium dioxide fumes, with a characteristic pungent odor, are liberated from a selenium rectifier when it burns out. The fumes should not be inhaled; therefore, ventilation of the instrument is of immediate importance. Replacement of the burned out rectifier should not be attempted until after it has cooled.

INSTRUCTIONAL ACTIVITIES

1. Demonstrate safety practices to be followed in working with electronic instruments. (As a first-period demonstration, this is an effective way of starting an electronics course.)
2. Demonstrate that a capacitor is not necessarily discharged in a de-energized circuit. Build a simple circuit containing a capacitor with no "bleeder" resistor connected to ground through which the capacitor can discharge. Energize the circuit for a brief time. After the circuit is de-energized, use a VOM or a CRT to show that a potential is stored on the capacitor.
3. Build a simple circuit in which a current of 100 mA lights a 0.1 A light bulb. After demonstrating this light bulb circuit, inform the students that 100 mA of current passing through the human body may be fatal.

PRACTICE PROBLEMS and STUDY QUESTIONS

1. The resistance of the body when wet is approximately 300 Ω. If a circuit is completed by a person simultaneously touching with each hand one of two points of differing potential, a current would flow hand-to-hand through that person's body. Calculate the potential difference required to cause a hand-to-hand current flow of:

    a.   1 mA
    b. 10 mA
    c. 100 mA

ANSWERS

1. a. 0.3 V
  b. 3 V
  c. 30 V

APPROACH TO SOLVING PROBLEMS

1. a. $E = IR = (1 \text{ mA})(300 \ \Omega) = 0.3$ V
  b. $E = IR = (10 \text{ mA})(300 \ \Omega) = 3$ V
  c. $E = IR = (100 \text{ mA})(300 \ \Omega) = 30$ V

CHAPTER 16

LOGICAL APPROACH TO TROUBLESHOOTING

The effectiveness of troubleshooting is determined largely by an operator's concentration and patience in applying good, sound common sense. Familiarity with an instrument's instruction manual and knowledge of instrumental operational principles, basic electronics, and the characteristic responses of problem-free instruments have direct relationships to the success of troubleshooting. The degree of comprehension of the principles of electronics and instrumentation is directly proportional to the level of detail with which a problem can be defined. The electrical engineer–instrument circuit designer should be able to pinpoint an instrumental problem to the specific malfunctioning circuit component. Persons of lesser electronic expertise may be able to isolate the cause of a malfunction to the general functional unit of the instrument. Technical personnel operating instruments in a laboratory should be able to determine at least this malfunctioning functional unit.

It has not been the intent of this book to discuss principles of operation of specific instruments. Therefore, this chapter on troubleshooting will not deal with specifics (except in the form of examples) but with the general logical approach to troubleshooting. The three main aspects of troubleshooting that will be discussed briefly are problem recognition, identification, and correction.

PROBLEM RECOGNITION

An instrument malfunction cannot be identified or corrected until it is apparent to the instrument operator that there is a problem. As basic and self-evident as this may seem, many malfunctioning instruments continue to produce inaccurate results because the instrument operators are not aware that a problem exists. Instrument malfunctions manifest themselves in many ways. Symptoms of instrument problems are sometimes very apparent and sometimes very subtle.

The accuracy of laboratory test results is jeopardized more by the subtle than by the readily apparent instrumental problems. Readily apparent problems include malfunctions that make a required analytical determination impossible, for example, a burned out light source in an optical counter, atomic absorption spectrophotometer, or spectrophotometer; a burned out galvanometer light bulb in a galvanometric readout in a spectrophotometer or osmometer; a blown fuse;

a ruined photodetector in any photometric instrument; depletion of fuels and/or reagents required for instrument function; or an unplugged power cord.

Problems expressed subtly require the alert, keen perception of an operator who is able to make fine distinctions between normal and abnormal instrument response characteristics. When these indistinctly expressed malfunctions are not detected, test result inaccuracies unfortunately may be accepted as valid. And therein lies the dangerous consequence of instruments being operated by poorly trained, unconscientious, unthinking robots. Examples of subtle malfunctions include: slight misalignment of the optical system in spectrophotometric instruments, dirty or damaged optical surfaces in optical analytical instruments, contamination of required fuels and/or solutions for instrument operation, damaged or worn electrical potentiometers, and alteration of reference voltages in potentiometric analytical instruments.

PROBLEM IDENTIFICATION

Once the effect of a problem is perceived, the cause or causes of that problem must be identified. Problem identification is, therefore, the matching of cause and effect. Experienced instrument operators may readily relate a specific faulty response to its cause because of the frequency with which they have previously observed that malfunction. The continued exposure of the operator to characteristic instrument responses and their identification produces a mental index of cause-effect relationships. (This index should be written out so that the less experienced may benefit.) Thus the expression "experience is the best teacher" applies to troubleshooting.

However, not all practicing technical laboratory personnel have this "index of experience" on which to rely. Therefore, each malfunction may be a new problem to solve. The apprehension of facing a new problem can be replaced gradually with the self-assurance that comes from being able to apply knowledge to problem solving in a logical, stepwise fashion. The familiarity of the problem solving approach diminishes or eliminates the uneasiness produced by the unknown.

The logical steps to be followed in troubleshooting are: state the perceived problem, list its possible causes (that is, formulate hypotheses), and then proceed to prove or disprove each hypothesis. Stating the problem caused by readily apparent malfunction is easy—for example, the light bulb went out in the spectrophotometer. More difficult are the subtle problems. These subtle problems present a constant challenge to the conscientious instrument operator. It is for identification of these malfunctions that persistent monitoring and vigilance are required. Calibration and quality control checks are the monitoring devices used for detection of subtle malfunctions or for forewarning of possible instrument problems. Preventive maintenance is a means of avoiding problems. Preventive maintenance procedures are well worth the time and effort invested, since the direct result is the avoidance of instrument problems that are detrimental to the speed and accuracy with which clinical laboratory analyses are performed. Calibration, quality control, and preventive maintenance are all too frequently approached with a "ho hum" attitude. However, these procedures are extremely important in indicating the presence of a subtle problem (for example, the warping of the photosensitive surface of a photovoltaic cell is best detected with a calibration check).

Possible causes of a problem should be listed in order of most to least probable. In the example of the spectrophotometer light bulb going out, the most probable cause would be a burned out bulb, followed by no current available to the bulb. The second possibility has a number of probable explanations: the power switch is off or the plug is not plugged into the power outlet (both of which are frequently responsible for inoperative instruments), a fuse is blown, the light bulb leads are not securely connected to the circuit connections, or no current is available from the power outlet. Additional causes of symptoms manifested by malfunctioning instruments are listed in most instrument operation manuals. If the most probable causes are proved not to be responsible for a problem, then these more comprehensive lists are very useful.

The procedure followed in proving or disproving hypothesized causes of a problem depends heavily upon common sense. In the example of the light bulb in the spectrophotometer, a quick visual check of the bulb will determine whether it is burned out. If the bulb is not burned out, further investigation is required. By observing whether other electrically operated parts of the circuit are functioning, the operator can determine whether the problem is limited to the bulb or has affected the entire circuitry of the instrument. (For example, if the "on-off" indicator light is on, a cooling fan is working, and the galvanometer light is on, then the problem is not a "no-power-to-the-circuit" problem.) If all electronic functions of the instrument are inoperative, then the following checks should be made: "on-off" switch in "on" position, power line plugged into power outlet, fuse not blown, and current available at the power outlet (check with a simple indicator light or a voltmeter, or ask an electrician). Frequently, one of these obvious, easily checked, probable causes is found to be responsible for the malfunction.

If all the obvious causes are eliminated as the responsible problem, additional circuit analysis procedures may be required. Even the electronics novice can visually check a circuit for melted, scorched, or damaged components. The odor of overheated components is also a good indicator of a problem within a circuit. Voltage and signal waveform checks require the use of an oscilloscope; voltage checks require only a voltmeter. Competence in the use of these test instruments and experience in obtaining electrical readings from circuits provide the needed expertise to follow the simple test point measurements given in many instrument manuals.

PROBLEM CORRECTION

Problem correction also should be the responsibility of the instrument operator. Two options are available. First, the operator may decide that the minor repair and/or replacement needed for correction of a malfunction is within his or her capabilities. Second, the operator may conclude that additional troubleshooting or malfunction correction requires additional expertise. With this conclusion, expert assistance should be obtained.

Of utmost importance is the expedient, effective repair of malfunctioning clinical laboratory instruments. The malfunction must be recognized and identified promptly. A judgment must be made as to the level of expertise required for its repair. And, finally, an honest evaluation of one's own abilities must be made to determine whether an expert should be called upon to correct the malfunction.

INSTRUCTIONAL ACTIVITIES

1. Set up troubleshooting exercises in a variety of instruments or circuits, requiring students to recognize, identify, and correct each instrument or circuit malfunction. For example, modify instruments or build simple circuits to include:
   a. A faulty potentiometer
   b. A faulty photovoltaic cell
   c. A faulty meter movement
   d. A deteriorating reference battery
   e. A lead containing a broken wire within the insulation
   f. A blown fuse
   g. A burned out light bulb
   h. A disconnected or loosely connected wire
   i. A faulty "on-off" switch

BIBLIOGRAPHY

Ackerman, Philip G. *Electronic Instrumentation in the Clinical Laboratory*. Boston: Little, Brown and Co., 1972.

Cromwell, Leslie; Arditti, Mort; Weibell, Fred J.; Pfeiffer, Erich A.; Steele, Bonnie; and Labok, Joseph A. *Medical Instrumentation for Health Care*. Englewood Cliffs, New Jersey: Prentice-Hall, Inc., 1976.

Diefenderfer, A. James. *Principles of Electronic Instrumentation*. Philadelphia: W. B. Saunders Co., 1972.

Ewing, Galen W. *Instrumental Methods of Chemical Analysis*. 4th ed. New York: McGraw-Hill Book Co., 1975.

Geddes, L. A., and Baker, L. E. *Principles of Applied Biomedical Instrumentation*. New York: John Wiley & Sons, Inc., 1968.

Graf, Rudolf F., ed. *Modern Dictionary of Electronics*. 3rd ed. Indianapolis: Howard W. Sams and Co., Inc., 1970.

Heath Co. *Understanding and Using Your Signal Generator*. Benton Harbor: Heath Co., 1963.

Hoenig, Stuart A., and Payne, F. Leland. *How to Build and Use Electronic Devices Without Frustration, Panic, Mountains of Money, or an Engineering Degree*. Boston: Little, Brown and Co., 1973.

Jacobowitz, Henry. *Electronics Made Simple*. New York: Doubleday and Co., Inc., 1965.

Jeffers, D. M., and Lowe, F. B. *Basic Electronics for Medical Technologists*. Houston: American Society for Medical Technology, 1971.

Karselis, Terence C. *Descriptive Medical Electronics and Instrumentation*. New Jersey: Charles B. Slack, Inc., 1973.

Lee, Leslie W. *Elementary Principles of Laboratory Instruments*. 2nd ed. Saint Louis: The C. V. Mosby Co., 1970.

Malmstadt, H. V.; Enke, C. G.; and Toren, E. C., Jr. *Electronics for Scientists*. New York: W. A. Benjamin, Inc., 1962.

Malmstadt, Howard V.; Enke, Christe G.; and Crouch, Stanley R. *Instrumentation for Scientists Series*. Module 1: *Electronic Analog Measurements and Transducers*. Reading, Massachusetts: W. A. Benjamin, Inc., 1973.

Mandl, Matthew. *Fundamentals of Electronics*. 3rd ed. Englewood Cliffs, New Jersey: Prentice-Hall, Inc., 1973.

Reilley, C. N., and Sawyer, D. T. *Experiments for Instrumental Methods*. New York: McGraw-Hill Book Co., 1961.

Skoog, Douglas A., and West, Donald M. *Principles of Instrumental Analysis*. New York: Holt, Rinehart and Winston, Inc., 1971.

Springer, John S. "Using Integrated Circuits in Chemical Instrumentation." *Analytical Chemistry* 42 (July, 1970): 22A–49A.

Strobel, Howard A. *Chemical Instrumentation: A Systematic Approach to Instrumental Analysis*. 2nd ed. Reading, Massachusetts: Addison-Wesley Publishing Co., 1973.

Tammes, A. R. *Electronics for Medical and Biology Laboratory Personnel*. Baltimore: The Williams and Wilkins Co., 1971.

White, Wilma L.: Erickson, Marilyn M.; and Stevens, Sue C. *Practical Automation for the Clinical Laboratory*. 2nd ed. Saint Louis: The C. V. Mosby Co., 1972.

Willard, Hobart H.; Merritt, Lynne L., Jr.; and Dean, John A. *Instrumental Methods of Analysis*. 4th ed. New York: Van Nostrand Reinhold Co., 1965.

Winstead, Martha. *Instrument Check Systems*. Philadelphia: Lea & Febiger, 1971.

Yanof, Howard M. *Biomedical Electronics*. 2nd ed. Philadelphia: F. A. Davis Co., 1972.

INDEX